SOTHIS PRESS

Sothis Press aims to completely reimagine the public domain book with an emphasis on universal access to captivatingly designed print editions. We believe that technology will enable every single book ever published to be perpetually accessible in beautiful print form. Sothis is beauty in ubiquity.

www.sothis.press
1 Waterhouse Square, London, ECIN 2ST

An Illustrated Repertory of Pains in Chest, Sides and Back

Their Direction and Character, Confirmed by Clinical Cases

Rollin R. Gregg

SOTHIS PRESS

ISBN 978-1-0368-0950-8

An Illustrated Repertory of Pains in Chest, Sides and Back is in the public domain.

ma-

J. E. Huffman
12-8-96

AN

Illustrated Repertory

OF

Pains in Chest, Sides and Back:

THEIR DIRECTION AND CHARACTER,

CONFIRMED BY

CLINICAL CASES.

By ROLLIN R. GREGG, M.D.

THIRD EDITION.

PREFACE.

This is the first instance, we believe, in the history of medicine, in which symptoms for medical guidance have been represented to the *sight;* and it becomes proper to consider what may be hoped for from it, in some other respects than those hereinafter named in the text.

Scientific men have always hitherto denied to medicine the position of a positive, or exact science; and with reason, because of its many uncertainties. But in view of all the facts herein pointed out, together with the order and system which we have endeavored to show can be given them, may we not hope to change their decision? Nature is ever true to herself, and our faith in her provision is unbounded. We believe that no limit will ever be found to the means she has provided to minister to the comfort, the welfare, and, the true happiness of the human race. The only difficulty is to find these and learn how to properly apply them. Whereever there is suffering to be relieved, there MUST be a remedy for it. It cannot be within the providence of God to be otherwise.

To avoid misunderstandings it seems to us proper to announce to the profession that, in view of the large expense we have already incurred in bringing our device, or plan, for representing symptoms, to its present state of development, we have felt compelled, as a matter of self-protection, to secure by copy-right, and by patent, this method of illustrating symptoms and the remedies for them, not only for Repertories and Materia Medicas, but for the various other uses to which it may be put in the advancement of medical science. There is no other way in which we could render ourselves secure in such an investment.

Having for several years fully tested the practical value of this Illustrated Repertory in the treatment of various diseases, and especially Consumption, it is now sent forth in book form, with the hope, that it may be of equal benefit to the whole profession as it has been to

THE AUTHOR.

BUFFALO, N. Y., March, 1879.

Contents.

CHAPTER V.

AN

Illustrated Repertory.

INTRODUCTION.

All know how greatly the study of anatomy, surgery, midwifery, and even of physiology, has been facilitated by means of figures and plates of the various parts and organs of the human body, and also of many of the natural operations transpiring within, or of the artificial operations performed upon it. Then why not make use of this same great aid in Therapeutics, where the knowledge which may be obtained thereby would be so much more important, because of so much more general use? The only question is, can such a work be properly done? This question we trust we shall be able to answer.

In this work is given the development of my plan for representing to the *eye* the pathogenetic symptoms of drugs, in a manner which furnishes, at the same view, the indications for their administration in disease. In other words an *Illustrated Repertory*, whereby we shall all be enabled to bring the powerful aid of the *sight* to the assistance of the other faculties, in determining by the locality, and the kind of symptoms, together with their direction and extent,—in all instances where they have these qualities,—that drug which is surely indicated in each individual case; and this without the necessity of that long and tedious search through several volumes, which is at present so often required to ensure the best success in the treatment of disease, by a strict application of the Homœopathic law.

It has long seemed to us impossible for any one to form in the mind, by reading alone, a clear and correct image of the full range of action of any one drug, and retain all its symptoms, especially if that drug has an extended action upon the system, and such a large number of symptoms as Aconite, Arsenicum, Belladonna, Mercurius, Sulphur, etc. At least we acknowledge our inability to do this. Detached portions of this image may be obtained and correctly impressed upon the mind, so that we can often make the proper application of the drug in the cure of the sick; but, we repeat, as to getting the whole image complete in all its parts, standing out in bold relief before the mind, ready for use under any and all circumstances, it seems to us impossible to be done by any means we have hitherto had to accomplish such a purpose. Yet, alas, what a terrible necessity exists for this being done. Then when we come to pass from one drug to the large number of these we use, the difficulties become multiplied just in proportion to numbers; while the mind becomes confused and memory literally overwhelmed with the vast multitude of symptoms which should, if they could, be retained.

These obstacles to those grand results which we know our system to be capable of, and which we are sure will ultimately always be attained, we must confess have been a source of serious trouble to us, individually, ever since we entered upon the practice of our profession. And the proving of more drugs has been adding to the confusion, notwithstanding the importance and need of these provings. Now, however, to our mind, much of this is changed, and we trust we do not build up false hopes to mislead others, when we claim that under the plan we present herein, a great portion of all this apparent confusion, comes out into that beautiful order and harmony which Nature everywhere displays, when we correctly interpret her language and accurately picture her work.

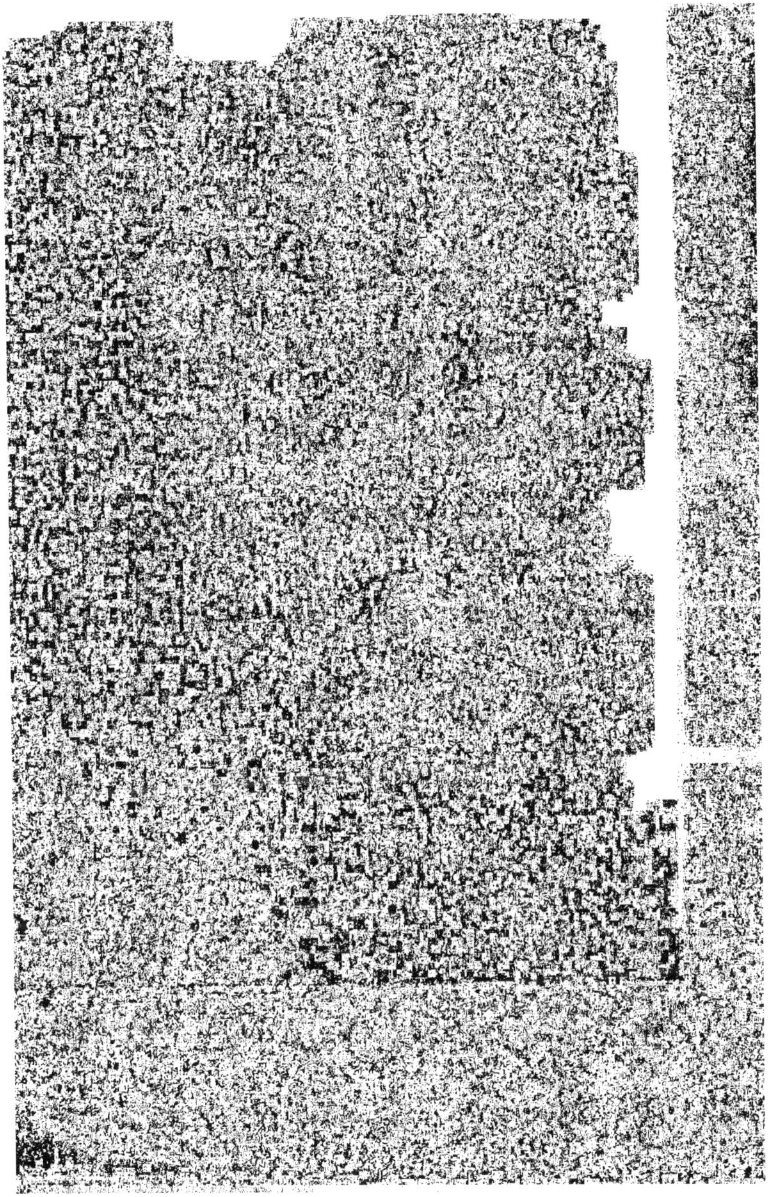

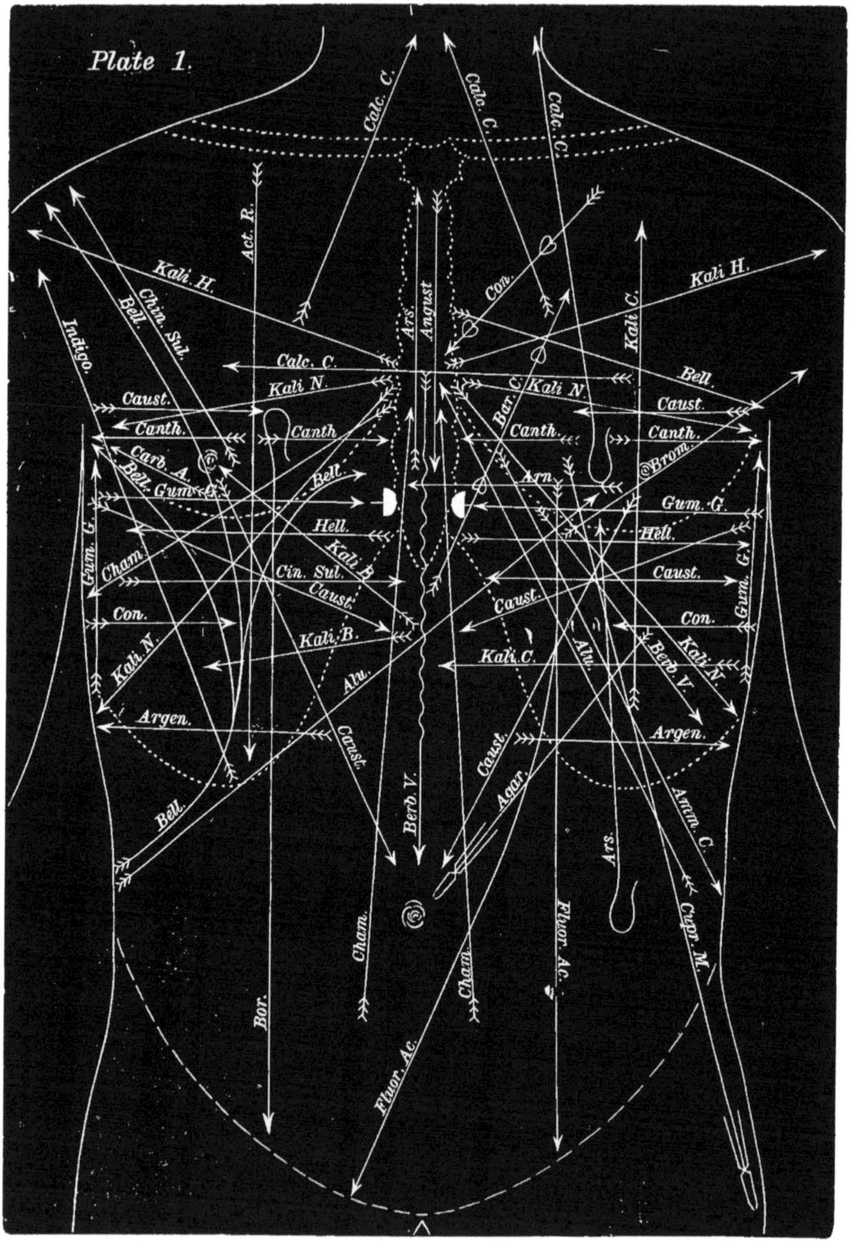
Plate 1.
Calc. C.
Calc. C.
Calc. C.
Act. R.
Kali. H.
Kali H.
Chin. Sul.
Bell.
Indigo.
Ars.
Angust
Con.
Kali C.
Calc. C.
Kali N.
Bar. C.
Kali N.
Bell.
Caust.
Caust.
Canth.
Canth
Canth.
Canth.
Carb. A.
Bell.
Gum. G.
Bell.
Arn.
Brom.
Gum. G.
Gum. G.
Hell.
Hell.
Kali B.
Cham.
Cin. Sul.
Caust.
Caust.
Caust.
Gum. G.
Con.
Con.
Kali. B.
Kali N.
Kali. C.
Alu.
Kali N.
Berb. V.
Alu.
Argen.
Argen.
Caust.
Caust.
Agar.
Bell.
Berb. V.
Amm. C.
Ars.
Cham.
Fluor. Ac.
Cupr. M.
Cham.
Bor.
Fluor. Ac.

CHAPTER I.

FRONT VIEW OF CHEST PAINS.

It is proposed now to give an illustration of chest pains chiefly, that are located in the front portion of the body.

These plates, as will be seen, have for their ground-work the outlines of the human body, from the neck to the hips. The arrows are used to indicate all the acute pains, such as *darting*, *stitching*, and the like, which pass from point to point in the chest, or from this to other parts of the body, and are placed upon the track of the pain; the tail upon the point where the pain arises, and the head where it terminates. The first two plates are intended for but one view of the chest, so that the tracks or lines of the arrows may be clearly traced without confusion; and also to afford room for the names of the drugs, which, in each instance, will be seen to be placed above, or immediately along-side, the arrow that represents its symptom. Where there are two heads upon an arrow, one at either end, it indicates darting, or stitching pains in *both* directions. The hook combined with the arrow signifies a *drawing* stitch, or a *drawing* ending in a stitch. The figure of a heart placed upon an arrow means a *throbbing* or *pulsating* stitch. The short lines or bars placed across the arrow signify a *tearing* stitch; they are to represent that if the arrow should move forward the bars would tear the tissues through which they passed. The pinchers stand for a *pinching* pain or a *pinching* stitch. The half-globe, or plano-convex figure, represents a *pressure* in connection with the stitching or darting pain. Where the line of the arrow is crooked it indicates a *contractive* stitch.

We will now give in detail the symptom, or symptoms, of each drug represented on the plates. These we copy direct from Hahnemann's Chronic Diseases, from the Symptomen Codex, and from Hull's Jahr's Symptomatology, as they are given there, and of course, as all these were procured by trials of the several drugs upon *well persons*, they are the characteristic symptoms which belong to the different ones respectively.

ACTEA RACEMOSA.

"Acute pain in the right lung, extending from apex to base, aggravated by respiration;" represented on plate 1 by the arrow correspondingly placed.

AGARICUS.

"Pinching in the left side of the chest down to the umbilicus;" illustrated by a pair of pinchers in the proper position.

ALUMINA.

"Lancination passing like lightning from the right loin to the left side of the chest, through the pit of the stomach when breathing;" and: "When stooping, a lancination coming out at the left side of the abdomen, and reaching the middle of the chest; the lancination comes on at every respiration; afterward, also, when standing straight."

AMMONIUM CARBONICUM.

Violent stitches in the left side of the chest, commencing in the præcordial region and then moving downward toward the side, and afterward toward the back.

ANGUSTURA.

Pressure across the whole right side of the chest and abdomen, as if these parts were compressed in front and behind, *accompanied* by an incisive cutting from above downward, in the sternum, and in the dorsal spine, increased by inspiration and every movement of the trunk.

ARGENTUM METALLICUM.

Violent cutting, in both sides, in the region of the lowest ribs, from within outward; the pain is severe only during a deep inspiration.

ARNICA.

Stitches in the heart, from the left side to the right, with fainting fits.

ARSENICUM ALBUM.

"Drawing-stitching pain under the left hypochondrium, extending into the chest when clearing the throat." This symptom is represented in plate 1 by the hook and arrow. Arsenicum album also has: "Stitching pain in the sternum from below upward, when coughing."

BARYTA CARBONICUM.

"Throbbing stitches in the left side of the chest, from the pit of the stomach upward;" represented by the arrow with two figures of a heart upon it.

BELLADONNA.

"Violent contractive griping in the right side of the abdomen when walking, accompanied by sharp stitches darting from that side through the right side of the chest and the axilla," as the Materia Medica has it, but we have considerable to add to this symptom from experience. Last summer we had a lady patient who was seized with a violent acute shooting pain, which started in at the right side of the abdomen, and extended up through the right side of the chest one branch of it shooting through to the vertebral border of the scapula, at a point about one-third of the distance upward from the inferior angle of this bone, and there causing the most extreme tenderness to touch; another branch of it extended to the right axilla, and a third branch of the pain extended to the top of the right shoulder. As would be expected from such a branching pain, there was, or seemed to be, much acute pain through all the lower half or two-thirds of the lungs besides, but these three branches predominated over all else, and stood out clear and distinct, while the suffering from them was, to all appearances, as great, if not greater than we ever before witnessed from acute pain. The lady had been an old chronic patient of ours for some three or four years, had suffered much from spinal irritation and very sensitive lungs for many years, was confined in May last, had several very severe chills, and two or three acute attacks of the lungs, threatening pleuro-pneumonia of a typhoid type, before she got up from her confinement. From all this she finally recovered sufficiently to be up about her house part of the time; but was left much emaciated, and with a severe cough and profuse purulent expectoration, night sweats, and much acute pain through the right lung; in fact had all the symptoms of phthisis so marked, that we were censured severely by some of her friends for giving encouragement of a cure in her case. Well, after continuing in this state a few weeks without much change, and no apparent relief of the acute pain from Aconite, Bryonia, Arsenicum, Phosphorus, etc., we were summoned to her one morning in haste, and found that the pain in the right lung had developed into the shooting, branching pain that we have described, and so violent was it, that she was almost suffocated from the obstruction to respiration, caused by its severity. The face was somewhat bloated and assuming a purplish hue, while the borders of the lips were already of a distinct purple. We at once prescribed Belladonna 2000, and visited her again in two hours, when we found her so much relieved that she could breathe quite comfortably, though of course the severe pain was not yet wholly controlled. She said she was very much relieved in the first half hour, while all appearances of threatened asphyxia had disappeared. From this on she recovered quite rapidly from cough, expectoration, and pain, though still, at times, suffering quite severely from the latter for some weeks, when more rapid improvement manifested itself, until she was restored to a better state of health, by September, than she had before enjoyed since a girl. And all this was done by Belladonna 2000, alone, without any other remedy.

Belladonna also has; "Fine stitches in the left side of the chest extending from the sternum toward the axilla, more violent during motion."

BERBERIS VULGARIS.

"Violent, sudden, incisive, contractive pain, in the front part of the middle portion of the chest extending down to the abdomen, obliging him to bend double;" represented in plate 1 by an arrow, the central portion of which is a crooked line, to give the idea of being contractive. This drug also has: "Painful dragging-sticking in the region of the heart, outward and downward."

BORAX.

Rivals Sepia in its stitching pains in the *right* lung, with this clear distinction, that the stitches of the former are many of them *drawing* stitches, while of the latter they are simply stitches; and with Borax; "The drawing stitches in the right side of the chest descend into the right groin, where he then feels a violent pain when hiccoughing, sneezing, coughing or gaping" These drawing stitches are represented by a hook, placed in about the centre of the right chest, and an arrow extending from it to the right groin.

BROMINE.

"Sticking pain in the left side of the chest toward the arm." The starting point of this pain not being given we place the arrow upon the track of a *drawing* pain through the left breast into the left arm, which is the preceding symptom of Bromine. Future experience must correct this if it is not right.

CALCAREA CARBONICUM.

"Stitches in the chest, toward the throat, for some hours;" represented by two arrows, one from each side, up into the throat. It also has: "Stitches across the chest, from the left to the right side, with a sensation as of constriction of the chest; his breathing was difficult, and during breathing the stitches became more violent;" and: "Stitches and drawing in the left half of the chest extending to the left submaxillary gland;" these being represented by a hook placed in the centre of the left chest, and an arrow extending from this up through the left side of the neck, as far as the figure allows.

CANTHARIS.

"Sticking pain and stitches in the chest, sometimes during an inspiration, in one or the other half of the chest, or one or the other side, extending to the axillæ, or into the sternum," represented by two arrows upon each side, one extending to the sternum and the other to the axilla.

CARBO ANIMALIS.

Stitches in the back part of the right breast, extending to the axilla.

CAUSTICUM.

"Sharp stitches in the chest, near the nipple, in the dircetion of the umbilicus, especially when breathing;" also: "Stitches in the outer parts of the chest, below the arm, extending to the pit of the stomach, accompanied by slight anguish;" all represented by two sets of arrows between the points named, though we suspect they are one and the same symptom differently expressed by different provers. Causticum also has: "Dull stitches from the axilla toward the chest," represented by the arrow in place upon *each* side, as no distinction is made in the language; and: "Sharp, slow stitches in the left side of the chest in a horizontal line with the pit of the stomach;" represented by a double headed arrow, as the direction is not given.

CHAMOMILLA.

"Stitches (rather dull) darting from the abdomen into the middle of the chest, as if caused by flatulence;" also: "Stitches from the middle of the chest to the right side after every inspiration."

CHININUM SULPHURICUM.

"Lancinations in the right half of the chest, extending toward the shoulder, arresting the breathing and relieved by bending the trunk forward; represented by an arrow extending from about the centre of the right lung up to the right shoulder.

CINCHONIUM SULPHURICUM.

"Stitches in the chest from the right side to the pit of the stomach."

CONIUM.

"Beating-stitch, with pain, in the upper and left part of the chest toward the centre of the chest;" represented by an arrow in the proper place, with two small figures of a heart upon it. Conium also has: "Violent stitches in the side, as if a knife were plunged into the side, causing loud moaning." Whether right or left, or both sides, is not here designated, so we place the arrow upon each side, and leave the matter for future confirmation or correction.

CUPRUM METALLICUM.

"Pinching pain in the left side of the chest extending to the hip;" represented by an arrow, in the proper place, with a pair of pinchers for its head.

FLUORIC ACID.

"Pain from the left side of the chest to the groin,

increased by deep respiration, particularly in the groin and back, like a stitch."

GUMMI GUTTI.

"Painful stitch from the ribs to the axilla, arresting the breathing;" whether upon one or both sides is not mentioned, but we place the arrow upon both, that experience may be had to settle the matter; and we give the direction perpendicularly beneath the axillæ, believing this to be the meaning of the symptom, though the language is ambiguous. Gummi gutti also has: "Pressure in the middle of the chest, and stitches going from both sides of the chest toward each other;" the pressure being represented in plate 1 by two plano-convex figures placed near the sternum, and the stitches, by the arrows coming from each side to them.

HELLEBORUS.

Sharp cutting in the region of the lowermost true ribs across the chest, from within outward, increased by inspiration.

INDIGO.

Painful spot, of the size of a hand, in the region of the right lower ribs, with a stitch extending to the shoulder joint when sitting (going off by motion.)

KALI BICHROMICUM.

"After dinner external stitches in the epigastrium and breast into the nipple (male), and in the right hypochondrium;" represented by two arrows running from the epigastrium, one to the right nipple, and the other to the right hypochondrium.

KALI CARBONICUM.

"Cutting sensation in the lower part of the chest, especially in the left side of it, moving into the epigastrium and leaving a stinging sensation in the left half of the chest," Kali carbonicum also produces: "Stitches under the left mamma, and sometimes ascending deep into the chest; also in the evening."

KALI HYDRIODICUM.

"Violent stitches in the middle of the sternum extending to the shoulder;" whether upon one or both sides is not named, so we carry the arrows to both shoulders in order to ensure future observation, and correct the error if it is one.

KALI NITRICUM.

"Stitches in the middle of the chest, extending to both sides and toward the axilla, when walking (during menses);" represented by two arrows upon each side, starting from the same point, and terminating, one in the axilla, the other at the lower part of the chest.

Since placing the arrows and writing the above, we have confirmed this symptom in a man, aged thirty-five years, an old and bad syphilitic subject, in whom the disease was suppressed, years ago, by Allopathic treatment. Dec. 13, 1869, he called upon us and said he had been suffering some weeks from severe acute pains in the chest, like the cutting of a knife. Upon inquiry for the exact locality of the pain, he placed the palm of his hand upon the centre of the sternum, and spreading the fingers said, "It shoots like that from the centre to the arm-pits and sides of the chest below, being about alike," he said "upon both sides." With this he had considerable cough and expectoration, and said he was feeling badly throughout his whole system. For these symptoms we prescribed Kali nitricum 3000, and he reported, the eighth day following, that by the fourth day after taking the medicine the pain was entirely relieved, and he was feeling much better in every way. Here, then, in this pain, is one of the great characteristics for this drug, independently of concomitants, for it will be borne in mind that this result was obtained upon the male organism, and, of course, was uninfluenced in any way by the menstrual function named in the quoted symptom above. And the symptom should be remembered as corresponding to several arrows upon each side, all starting from behind the centre of the sternum and radiating from thence, the upper one to the axilla, and the others from this along down to the lower ribs upon each side.

This completes all the remedies represented in plate 1, and we now pass to plate 2.

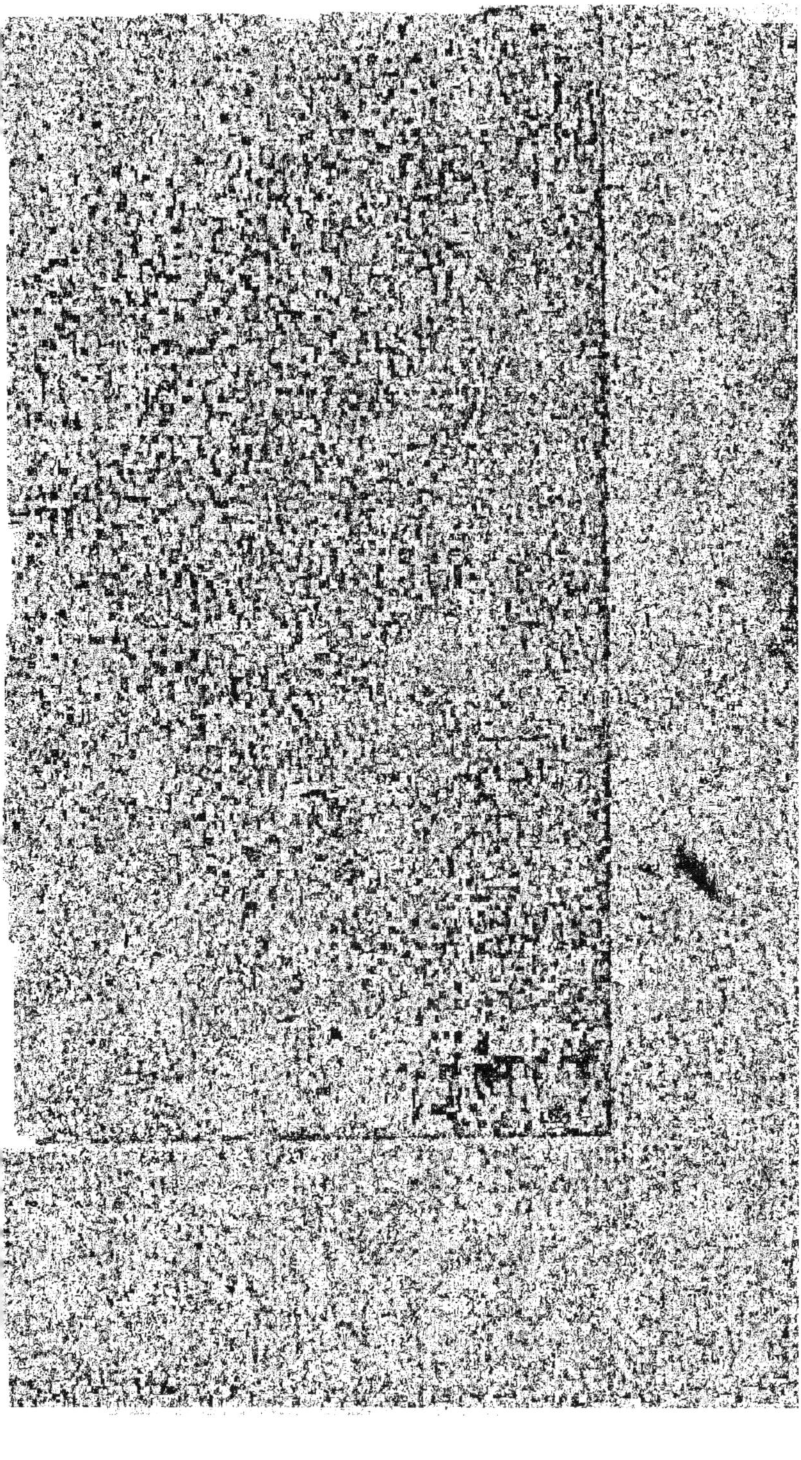

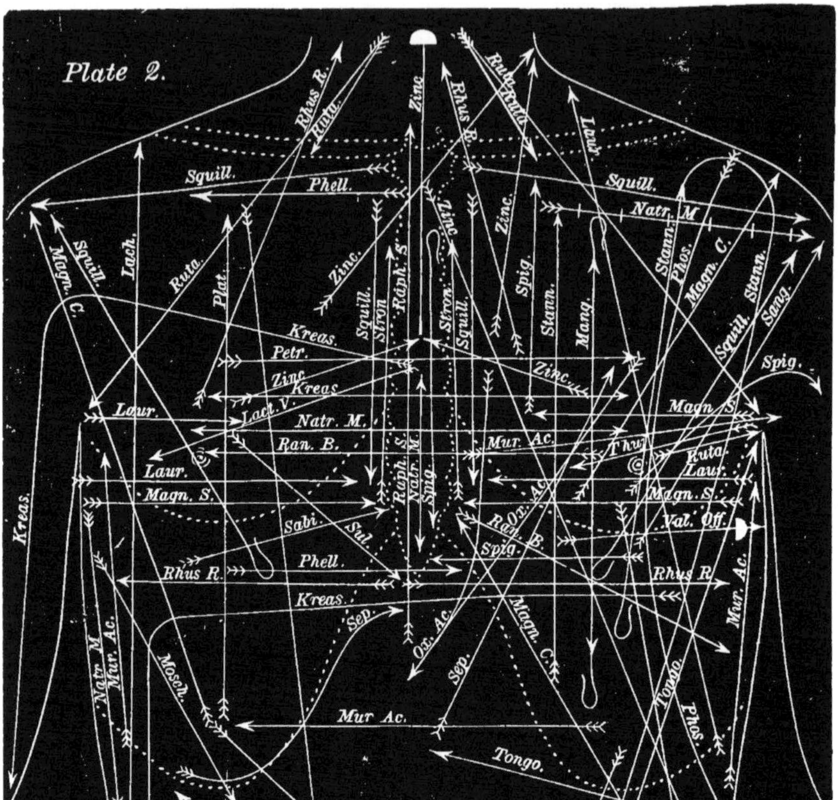
Rhus R.
Ruta.
Zinc.
Rhus R.
Ruta.
Ruta.
Laur.
Squill.
Phell.
Squill.
Natr. M.
Magn. C.
Squill.
Lach.
Ruta.
Plat.
Zinc.
Squill.
Stron.
Raph. S.
Zinc.
Stron.
Squill.
Zinc.
Spig.
Stann.
Mang.
Stann.
Phos.
Magn. C.
Squill.
Stann.
Sang.
Spig.
Kreas.
Petr.
Zinc.
Kreas.
Zinc.
Lact. V.
Laur.
Natr. M.
Magn. S.
Ran. B.
Mur. Ac.
Thuj.
Ruta.
Laur.
Laur.
Magn. S.
Magn. S.
Raph. S.
Natr. M.
Spig.
Ox. Ac.
Val. Off.
Sabi.
Sul.
Ran. B.
Spig.
Phell.
Rhus R.
Rhus R.
Kreas.
Mur. Ac.
Kreas.
Sep.
Ox. Ac.
Sep.
Magn. C.
Natr. M.
Mur. Ac.
Mosch.
Tongo.
Phos.
Mur. Ac.
Tongo.
Magn. C.
Zinc.
Rhus T.
Nit. Ac.
Lach.
Stann.
Phos. Ac.
Sep.
Kreas.

Plate 2.

KREASOTUM.

"Acute stitches in the middle of the chest, worse during an inspiration, attended with a feeling of lameness, and extending to the elbow joint across the right shoulder, where the pains are most violent on lifting the arms." This symptom, Dr. L. M. Kenyon, of this city informs us he has confirmed in two cases, one some ten or twelve years since, the other more recent; that it occurred in both as a concomitant of *chronic leucorrhœa* and that both were very promptly relieved by Kreasotum. This drug also produces: "Stitches below the left mamma, proceeding thence as with a sharp knife, and like an electric shock across the pit of the stomach, the chest, the right side of the abdomen, thighs, down to the tarsal joints." Each of these symptoms is represented by its appropriate arrow, with the head of it carried in each case as far as the size of our plate will allow. The same drug further has: "Sticking across the middle of the chest from morning till noon," which, as the direction is not given, we represent with a double headed arrow, as though the pain passed both ways, and thus leave it for future experience to correct, if it is wrong.

LACHESIS.

"Stitch through the chest, from the abdomen to the shoulder;" as expressed under the chest symptoms, but explained under the abdominal symptoms as follows; "Stitches from the right os ilium, through the abdomen and chest, as far as the shoulder; after which the stitches strike from the left lower to the right upper side" of the abdomen, we infer, and place this arrow accordingly.

LACTUCA VIROSA.

Pleuritic stitches from the middle of the sternum toward the right side.

LAUROCERASUS.

"Stitches through both sides of the chest toward the sternum;" and: "Stitches from the right axilla to the chest." It also produces: "Stinging tension in the left side when lying on it, extending up to the neck, in the morning."

MAGNESIA CARBONICA.

"Stitches below the right side of the chest, toward the umbilcus, or darting out at the shoulder, also during an inspiration;" and: "Dull stitches in the left half of the chest, during an inspiration, extending into the shoulder." Magnesia carbonica also produces: "Stitches below the left half of the chest, when yawning, also after dinner, or in the evening when they are felt in a sitting posture, and sometimes extend into the sternum."

MAGNESIA SULPHURICA.

"Stitches from either side toward one another, in the evening, on entering the room from the open air;" and: "Stitches from the left axilla to the chest.".

MANGANUM.

"Drawing-stitch in the left half of the chest, darting continually upward and downward;" represented in plate 2 by a hook and arrow-head at each end of the arrow, and this placed perpendicularly in the left chest. This drug also produces: "A sticking pain in the chest from below upward, which is sometimes felt during an expiration;" which we cannot locate from this language, so we do not represent it on the plate.

MOSCHUS.

Stitches in the right side, down to the region of the liver.

MURIATIC ACID.

"Tensive darting from the left false ribs to the right ribs;" also: "Stitches deep in the præcordial region, extending as far as the axilla and back, with stitches in the thigh extending to the knee, when sitting, going off when rising." Muriatic acid also produces: "Slowly ascending, broad stitches, externally in the sides of the chest."

NATRUM MURIATICUM.

"Stitching pain, transversely through the lungs, in frequent attacks, at intervals of an hour;" represented by an arrow with a head upon each end; and: "Single stitches along the sternum;" which, as the direction is not given, is also represented by a double headed arrow. Natrum muriaticum produces also: "Tearing stitching pain from the left upper region of the chest to the shoulder-joint;" represented by an arrow with bars across it; and: "Dartings under the right arm down the side."

NITRIC ACID.

Violent stitch, in the upper part of and within the right ribs, through the abdomen and back.

NUX MOSCHATA.

"Darting in the fore part of the chest, shooting upward in an oblique direction and arresting the breathing;" not represented on the plate by an arrow, as the locality is not given definitely enough to locate it, but mentioned here so that future experience will be had to properly locate it.

OXALIC ACID.

Sharp shooting pain in the left lung and heart, extending down to the epigastrium, lasting for some seconds.

PETROLEUM.

"Lancinating pain, in front, from the right to the left side of the chest, when bending the trunk to the left side." It also has: "Violent stitch as far as the heart, arresting the breathing;" which we cannot locate, as the point of its origin is not named.

PHELLANDRIUM AQUATICUM.

"Pointed stitch in the upper part of the sternum, somewhat to the right;" also: "Dull stitches from the last true rib to the xiphoid cartilage, with painful sensation in the stomach, as if screwed together." The side not being mentioned in this instance, we place the arrow upon the right side, to correspond with a similar pain given under the abdominal symptoms, and thus located.

PHOSPHORUS.

Very violent stitching pains, starting in just beneath the skin upon the acromial extremity of the left clavicle, and shooting from there downward through the left lung, and out at the left side of the abdomen, just below the ribs. This is not from the Materia Medica, as there are no acute pains passing from point to point, given there under Phosphorus, which can be represented by a front view of the chest; but is a symptom which we recently found by clinical experience to be readily controlled by this drug. The case here follows: We were called to a tall powerful man having this symptom in great severity. After laboring under a severe cold a week or ten days, he was taken very suddenly with this pain, was in a severe chill at the time of our call, and apparently under extreme suffering. There was utter inability to take any but the shortest inspirations; great aggravation upon the slightest movement of the body; and it was impossible for him to lie upon the left side. Though there is no drug in the Materia Medica covering this symptom, we prescribed Phosphorus 3000, with confidence and awaited results. The next day we found the chill had been soon relieved, and the pain greatly mitigated within two or three hours, when a profuse perspiration broke out and put an end to further suffering from pain. And early that morning he commenced expectorating very thick, heavy, yellow sputa, which was accompanied with considerable blood; so the pain was from no mere neuralgic action that would soon have subsided of itself. The expectoration almost wholly ceased in the course of that forenoon, a gentle perspiration continued some two or three days, and the patient rapidly convalesced without any other remedy. Now, believing this speedy and marked relief have been due to a specific and powerful action of Phosphorus, we place the arrow, to represent the symptom, upon plate 2, with confidence in its value for future guidance in cases where there is suffering from like pains, similarly located.

PHOSPHORIC ACID.

Dull stitch in the left side between the lowest rib and the pelvis, through the whole cavity of the abdomen, more violent during an inspiration.

PLATINA.

Cutting shocks in the right chest from below upward.

RANUNCULUS BULBOSUS.

"Sticking in the side of the sternum toward the left side, with sensation as if bruised, while going up hill." It also produces: "Pain" which "extends from the left into the right chest, the sticking pain being felt in both sides of the chest at the same time, however he is able to take deep breath while bending forward.

RAPHANUS SATIVUS.

Pain in the chest, particularly when eating and coughing, less when drinking, the pain being of an aching and sticking character, extending from the pit of the stomach to the throat-pit, and frequently to the back.

RHUS RADICANS.

"Stinging-tearing pain in the sides of the chest, commencing in the stomach, and extending first to the left side of the chest, then to the right;" and: "In the forenoon when walking, sharp pain in the left side of the chest, feeling as if it extended to the throat;" is also has: "Painful stitches in the right side of the chest, extending to the neck, aggravated by motion and deep inspiration."

RHUS TOXICODENDRON.

Lancination from the left chest to the left side of the abdomen (in the evening).

RUTA GRAVEOLENS.

"Sharp stitches between the left nipple and axilla, more violent during an inspiration;" also: "Fine cutting, which extends from the throat into the chest, especially into the region of the clavicle and the axilla, where it stops; the cutting is felt when walking, and becomes worse as one walks faster." The side not being given in this last instance, we place the arrows upon both sides, subject to confirmation, or correction, if one is wrong.

SABÍNA.

Sharp stitches in the region of the last true ribs of the right side, toward the sternum, only during an inspiration.

SANGUINARIA.

Stitches from the lower part of the left breast to the shoulder.

SEPIA.

"Stitch around the right lower rib, toward the pit of the stomach, continuing for minutes, going off by an empty eructation;" and: "Stitches darting occasionally from the epigastrium close below the pit of the stomach into the left side, upward;" also: "Stitches from the umbilicus to the genital organs, when coughing and throwing off mucus."

SPIGELIA.

"Lancinating pain commencing below the left nipple, and

extending into the region of the scapula, and upper arm, more violent during deep inspirations." That part of this symptom relating to the arm is represented in plate 2 by its appropriate arrow, while that which extends to the scapula will be given in a side view. Spigelia also produces: "Sudden, drawing, stinging pain along the sternum from above downward;" represented by the hook and arrow properly placed. This drug further produces: "Momentary, violent sticking pain in the left chest toward the clavicle, preventing the breathing, in the evening;" and: "Dull oppressive sticking in the heart, between the region where the beats of the heart are felt, and the scrobiculus cordis; the same sticking is felt, in and above the scrobiculus cordis, and the chest is oppressed."

SQUILLA MARITIMA.

"Drawing stitch from the last true rib as far as the shoulder;" which, as the language is so indefinite, we represent upon both sides, and leave the future to correct one, if wrong. This drug further has: "Pointed stitches in the region of the extremity of the clavicle toward the shoulder, during an inspiration and expiration;" and: "Excessive stitching near the sternum from above downward, making the breathing difficult;" which are also represented upon both sides.

STANNUM.

"Sudden drawing under the left breast when raising one's self in the bed, followed by sharp cuttings extending thence to the clavicle, in the direction of the shoulder where the pain remains fixed; thence it moves along the left shoulder into the abdomen, made worse when drawing in the chest, pressing upon the part, and especially during an inspiration and vomiturition; in all these conditions the pain is felt as a painful jerk." Stannum also has: "Frequent cuttings through the chest from below upward, and in front in the region of the upper ribs from within outward, independent of breathing." This we suspect may be a repetition of the previous symptom, given in different language by another prover, so we represent it only upon the left side, but in this may be wrong.

STRONTIANA CARBONICUM.

Shootings through the chest, from below upward, along both sides of the sternum.

SULPHUR.

"Violent stitches from the right chest through the pit of the stomach and the stomach;" and: "Cutting in the chest down to the pit of the stomach;" both of which, it seems to us, must be meant for one symptom, so we represent them with one arrow upon the right side.

THUJA.

Strong, dull, intermittent stitches in the chest, from the left axilla inward.

TONGO.

"Stitches under the left chest extending to the axilla;" and: "Bruised sensation and cutting under the left chest, thence shifting to the pit of the stomach and back again, relieved by pressure."

VALERIANA OFFICINALIS.

Dull stitch, resembling a pressing from within outward, in the left side of the chest (below the axilla), during a deep inspiration: the stitch lasts as long as the inspiration.

ZINCUM METALLICUM.

"Violent stitches in the chest when walking in the open air, extending as far up as the left side of the neck, with difficult breathing for several hours." The wording of this leads us to infer the stitches must pass up from both sides of the chest, and we so represent it. Zincum also has: "Violent stitches into the sternum when stooping, followed by painful pressure extending from the inmost chest into the throat." All this is represented by a pair of arrows, one from each side, extending into the centre of the sternum and a line continuing from thence up to the throat, where a plano-convex figure is placed to represent the pressure. This drug further has: "Stitch in the upper part of the sternum, extending into the left lumbar region, with dread of stooping early in the morning."

This closes the list of the older and more reliable remedies for those diseases that have acute pains passing from point to point in the chest, which can be represented by a *front* view of this portion of the body. There are several of the remedies having a place on the plates that have darting, stitching, or kindred pains, in addition to those given, which we are left to infer, from the language, extend a longer or shorter distance in the chest, but which, unfortunately, we cannot represent, as the origin and termination are not given, nor the lung in which they occurred. There are also others not given on the plates, that have the same kind of pains, evidently extending from one point to another in the chest; but neither point being named, we have been compelled to omit them, much to our regret and annoyance. The terms "long lancinating pains," "long stitches," and "stitches darting through the chest," occur under several drugs, without the track they traverse being named in any way so that the arrow could be located. The only remedy now for this serious defect in the re-proving of all such medicines, and accurately giving the exact localities of these symptoms, with the points of their origin and termination distinctly named in each instance; and we regard it as important that this should be done. While upon this part of our subject, we will also call upon all provers of drugs in the future, to name accurately the exact point, or points, of the body, upon or beneath which the symptoms appear; if posterior to a rib, for instance, state by number which rib, and the exact place upon it behind which the symptom occurs; the direction and extent of all symptoms where they have these qualities, or their exact origin and termination; and by all means the side of the body, or the limb, whether right or left, or both, in which the symptoms occur. Rigid care in the future upon these and all like matters, will be of incalculable value to the profession and to mankind.

There are still other instances than those above named, where stitching and kindred pains occur, either in succession, or alternation, in different parts of the chest, or now in the chest, then in the stomach, abdomen, groins, shoulders, etc., while they do not exist, or pass *between* these points; and these are not given on the plates now represented, as the arrow would not correctly represent them.

It will have been seen that on the plates, and in the symptoms quoted from the various drugs, we have both represented and used the words acute, cutting, darting, incisive, lancinating, piercing, stabbing, sharp, shooting, sticking, stinging, etc., synonymously, and given the arrow to represent each indiscriminately, because patients will not certainly discriminate, and many of them cannot, between these various words, and use them literally according to their true meaning: one using one of the words, and another selecting another word of similar meaning to convey the same symptom, just as each should be most familiar with the word he used. We doubt if even educated physicians would not use, some one, and some another of the above-named words to express the pain. Indeed, by reading the Materia Medica closely, it will be seen that most of these words are there used synonymously. For instance, stitches darting so and so, or lancinating pains, shooting so and so, etc., are common expressions.

Far above and beyond all else, it is unnecessary to make any distinction between these various but similar pains, for there is a fact in connection with this very point, brought out by illustrating symptoms in this way, which shows clearly that there is no need for any distinction. Nature evidently provided against any necessity for it, and against the errors which would certainly be committed by different persons, endeavoring to distinguish by the uncertain medium of language, between certain pains, which by name are different, and yet have so great a similarity. This fact, so brought out, which surprised us and no doubt will surprise others, is this: Though the plates may, at first view, appear somewhat complicated or confused, yet among all the drugs thus far proved and represented thereon, there are but very few of them in which the arrows that represent their symptoms, even seem to conflict with each other, by extending between the same points; and no two where the symptoms are exactly alike, or, indeed, where the language of the symptoms is not sufficiently distinct, in itself, to point out a clear difference, while the concomitants will make the matter doubly sure and allow of no mistake as to the drug indicated.

To illustrate this, we will take up some of the drugs represented, whose symptoms seem to clash. Gummi gutti, Laurocerasus and Magnesia sulphurica each have a pair of arrows, one upon either side, extending from the sides of the chest toward each other, and to near the sternum, and in this bare fact there is no difference; but let us look a little more closely into the matter. Gummi gutti has: "*Pressure in the middle of the chest*, and stitches going from both sides of the chest toward each other," represented in plate 1 by the figure we have chosen to illustrate pressure, placed one upon either side of the sternum, and the arrows running toward them; while with neither Laurocerasus, nor Magnesia sulphurica, is there any mention of pressure at any point in connection with the stitches. This certainly makes a clear and marked distinction, and takes the former, or Gummi gutti, out of the list for comparison, and destroys the appearances of real similiarity in symptoms. The difference between Laurocerasus and Magnesia sulphurica is not so decided in this one symptom, however, and yet there is a clear distinction as seen by the following. Magnesia sulphurica has: "Stitches trom either side toward one another, *in the evening on entering the room from the open air;*" while Laurocerasus has simply: "Stitches through both sides of the chest toward the sternum," without reference at all to the evening, or entering the room from the open air, and this makes a clear distinction certainly, and one that is sufficient. But nature, as if fearful of being caught at fault upon this point, has added a most positive distinction between the two drugs, in their stitching pains in the chest, for she gave to Laurocerasus the power to produce and cure "Stitches from the *right* axilla to the chest," and to Magnesia sulphurica the power to both cause and cure "Stitches from the *left* axilla to the chest," making the two the exact antipodes of each other in this respect.

Chamomilla and Lactuca are two other remedies which seem to conflict, yet do not. Chamomilla has: "Stitches from the middle of the chest *to* the right side, *after every inspiration;*" while Lactuca has: "Pleuritic stitches from the middle of the sternum *toward* the right side," without any reference to inspiration in connection with this symptom.

And the concomitants of these symptoms are as different under the two drugs as it is possible for them to be. For instance, with Chamomilla the condition of the throat and larynx are characteristically those arising from a free secretion of mucus in these parts, causing rattling respiration; and "almost uninterrupted titillation under the *upper part of the sternum;*" with Latuca on the contrary, the prominent feature is "*roughness*" and "*dryness*" of those parts, and "*dry* cough," and "cough from tickling in the *throat.*" Again, the great characteristic features of the chest symptoms under the latter remedy are, "*oppression* of," and "*heaviness* on the chest," as if oppressed by a great weight, while with Chamomilla these symptoms have no prominence, in fact oppression is but barely mentioned, and heaviness not at all named under its chest symptoms.

Calcarea carbonicum and Ranunculus bulbosus, are two other remedies which seem to rival each other upon the plates, in the fact that each has an arrow extending from the *left* into the *right* side of the chest, to represent "*stitches*" with the former, and "*sticking*" with the latter drug, passing in that direction; but with Ranunculus bulbosus, the sticking pain is felt in *both* sides at the *same time,*" which is not a condition of the stitches of Calcarea. But to make assurance doubly sure, Nature was again on the alert, in the fact that she gave to Calcarea the characteristic symptom, "difficult breathing, relieved by bending (or drawing) the shoulders backward;" but with Ranunculus bulbosus the conditions are just the opposite, the patient being "able to take a deep breath while bending forward," and "he has to sit or stand stooping with his head and chest forward." Again Calcarea has this: "The breath becomes short when *ascending the least height,*" which is a leading characteristic of this drug; under Ranunculus bulbosus, on the contrary, all of this is exactly reversed, as shown in the following: "Pressure in the chest, and shortness of breath when walking on the level ground, but *no oppression* of breathing when *going up hill.*"

And so it is with the few remaining remedies that have arrows upon the plates, which seem to conflict by passing in the same direction, and between the same points; they could be shown to be so different in most of their other symptoms, and so directly opposite in some, that no mistake could be made as to which was indicated for this one similar symptom; but we have neither the time nor the space to draw the comparison, and therefore must throw the labor of it upon the reader, who can do it as well as we, now that he has the key by which it should be done. But with the great majority of the remedies represented on the plates, there is no confusion caused by the position of the arrows; and it is curious to see how exactly opposite some are in their direction with reference to others, and how entirely different a few are in their location, direction, and extent, from all the rest. When we commenced this work we had no expectation of finding what we have, supposing there would be a great similarity in many of the remedies, with reference to the location and direction of the arrows, but thought that by representing the symptoms to the eye, we could all get, upon the whole a better idea of the various drugs and their range of action, and this was all we hoped for. Therefore our surprise at what we did obtain, may be better imagined than expressed.

Another remarkable feature, as it appears to us, which has been developed by this method of illustrating symptoms, is the fact that the stitching pains, which are caused and cured by the various drugs, few or none of them pass along the lines of nerves or the fibres of other tissues, for neither the nerves or other tissues have continuous fibres passing in that direction, and to the distance, that such stitches frequently do. In our casual reflections hitherto upon this part of our subject, but without giving it careful study, we had supposed, as a matter of course, that all acute pains must, of necessity pass along the filaments of some nerve or nerves, for a longer or shorter distance of their course, in a direction outwardly from the nervous centres, or inwardly toward these; or that they might pass along the filaments of fibrous tissues, and here we supposed was the limit and guide to all such symptoms; but see how far this was from the truth. Take the symptom of Belladonna, for instance, which we have represented as extending from the right side of the abdomen by three lines, upward through the right chest; there are no continuous filaments of nerves or any other tissues passing such a distance, in those directions. Again, Kreasotum shows an equal independence of continuous fibres of tissues upon which to travel, in its stiches shooting from below the left breast across to the right side of the chest, and down through the right side of the abdomen and the leg into the toes. The same may be said also of Stannum in its drawing stitches, shooting upward through the left chest to the clavicle, and there turning and darting downward again into the abdomen; and of Phosphorus, with its stitching pain from the point of the left shoulder down through the left lung and out at the left side of the abdomen. There are no continuous fibres of any of the tissues passing in these various directions, and to such extent, upon which the pains could travel; but instead of this, they strike through and across all classes of tissues indiscriminately, without guide or regard for the structures over or through which they pass.

To our mind this shows more clearly and forcibly the specific action and power of drugs, than anything else in connection with their effects upon the human organism, and must it not be, that this fact, taken in connection with the other that these results are, most of them, in appearance, and all, in fact so different from each other, when we come to portray them to the eye, must not all this, we repeat, raise these hitherto, perhaps, too much neglected symptoms into prominent if not leading characteristics? And does not all this give us a reliance upon our Materia Medica that we could not have without? We have heard much in times past, and read some articles, charging that many of the symptoms of the drugs, given as provings, were imaginary, or not the specific effect of medicine; and no doubt some in our school entertain this view now, while all in the old school, who have any knowledge upon the subject, so regard them. It is no doubt within the province and power of the imagination for it to excite nausea in some persons, who should attempt to prove drugs, especially where they had previously been greatly nauseated by medicine; or possibly to cause, in others, gripings in the abdomen, if they had previously taken active cathartics; but no extent or stretch of imagination could excite, or in any way lead to, such stitching pains as we have illustrated as the effect of medicines, and so different with each drug from that of any of the rest. Nor is it possible for them to be accidental. Instead of either of these, the results, when viewed in this light, show for themselves, that they belong in each instance to the drug that is credited with them, and to nothing else; in other words, that they are *specific*. And do not these great facts, taken either individually or collectively, show the mistake in alternating remedies?

In quoting the symptoms, it will be seen that we have not made the distinctions, by italics, as is done in the Materia Medica. This appeared to us unnecessary, as the symptoms are really so different when represented to the eye. It should also be understood, that the symptoms we represent on the plates, are all copied from among the chest symptoms under the various drugs, excepting in a few instances where we have made use of the stomach, or abdominal symptoms, to correct or explain the others. When this work comes to be extended to illustrate the shooting pains of the hypochondria, the stomach, and the abdomen, it will be seen that many of these reach into various parts of the chest. And the same may be said of the darting pains of the throat and neck. Many of them will be found to descend into the chest.

It seems unnecessary to dwell upon the advantages of this method of representing symptoms, for they must be apparent to all. The two plates illustrate, certainly, not less than from three hundred to four hundred pages, which we have read, from which to select the symptoms, and all of which every physician is liable to have to read for each case with any like symptoms, to gather these by the old method, for application at the bed-side; with the certainty of his forgetting many, if not the most of them, among the multiplicity of his professional duties. Even those symptoms now illustrated, when separated from all else, and placed by themselves, would fill some eleven pages of fine print, and we doubt if there are many in the profession who can commit them to memory, without the aid of the plates, and retain them for use, to say nothing of the great number of other symptoms he needs to remember. But the plates will make all this part of his labor unnecessary, and leaves him free to apply his mind to such symptoms as cannot be illustrated.

Chapter II.

VIEW OF PAINS OF RIGHT SIDE.

We continue our work in this chapter, by giving a view of the right side of the body, for the darting or stitching pains of the chest and back, which can be represented by such a view. We have added two characters not given in the previous plates. One of these stands for a symptom, and will in the future always be used, when occasion requires, to illustrate any similar symptoms; the other may be said to stand for a fact in connection with some of the symptoms. The former is a figure of one of the forms of a flame from a jet of gas, and is to be understood now, as representing *burning* pains; or when placed upon the arrow as is the case on the accompanying plate, to illustrate a symptom of Oleum animale in the upper right chest, it means a *burning* stitch. The character given to represent a fact in connection with some symptoms, is that of a small *circle*, with two or more arrows running out from the centre of this, and shows that in such cases the symptoms start from a common centre, or have a common point of origin.

There has been much more difficulty in representing symptoms by a side view, than there was in a front view of the chest, in order to give the correct idea of their exact origin and termination, for the reason that we have to give upon an entirely flat surface what so peculiary belong to a rounded one. For instance, a symptom starting from under the mamma, and passing through to any part of the back, to have its arrow correspondingly placed, may look, upon first

Plate 3.

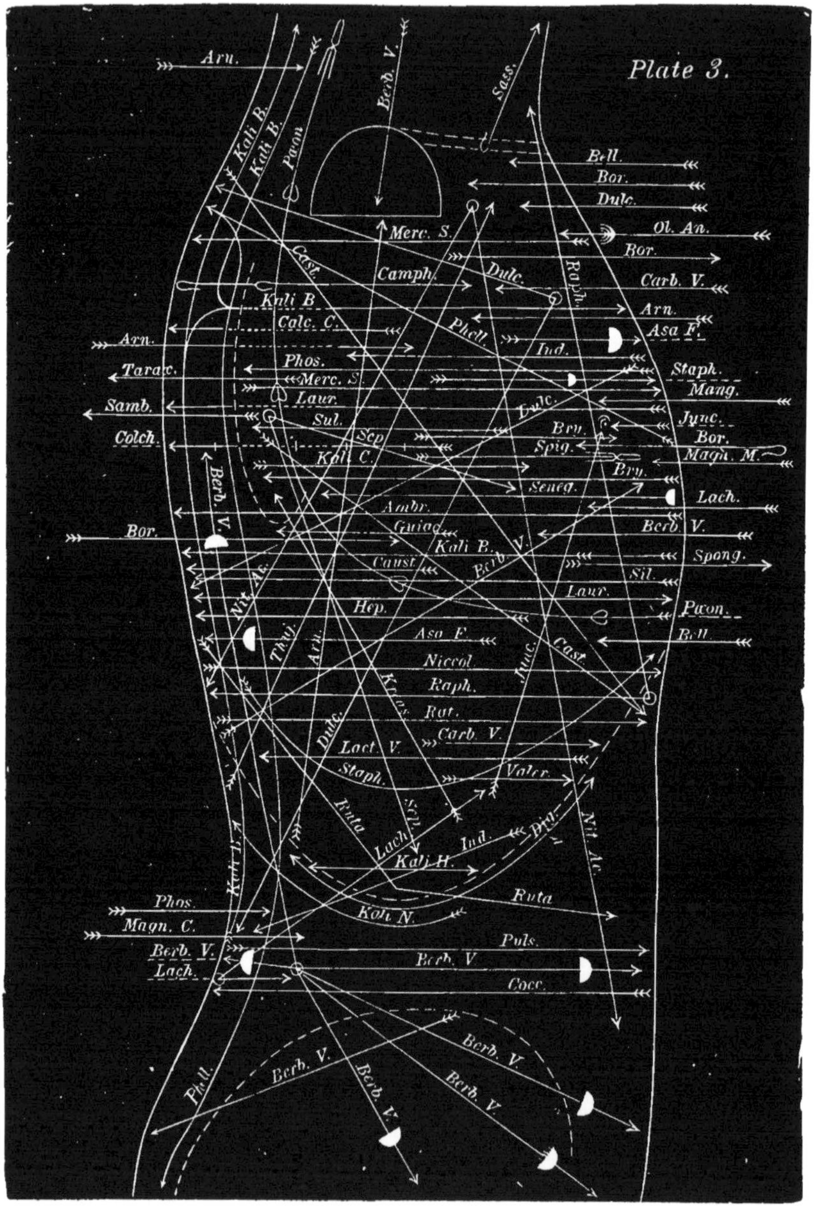
Arn.
Berb. V.
Sass.
Kali B.
Kali B.
Pæon
Bell.
Bor.
Dulc.
Merc. S.
Ol. An.
Bor.
Cast.
Camph.
Dulc.
Raph.
Carb. V.
Kali B
Arn.
Calc. C.
Phell.
Asa F.
Arn.
Ind.
Phos.
Staph.
Tarax.
Merc. S.
Mang.
Laur.
Samb.
Dulc.
Junc.
Sul.
Bor.
Sep.
Bry.
Colch.
Spig.
Magn. M.
Kali C.
Bry.
Seneg.
Berb. V.
Lach.
Ambr.
Guiac.
Berb. V.
Bor.
Kali B.
Spong.
Caust.
Berb. V.
Sil.
Nit. Ac.
Laur.
Hep.
Pæon.
Thuj.
Arn.
Asa F.
Bell.
Niccol.
Junc.
Cast.
Raph.
Rut.
Dulc.
Carb. V.
Lact. V.
Staph.
Valer.
Ruta
Nit. Ac.
Lach.
Ind.
Kali H.
Ruta
Kali N.
Phos.
Magn. C.
Puls.
Berb. V.
Berb. V.
Lach.
Coce.
Berb. V.
Phell.
Berb. V.
Berb. V.
Berb. V.

view, as though it started at a point some depth in from the front wall of the chest, and so of any symptom starting from any point on the surface of the chest, out from the median line of the sternum, or upon the back from any point to the right of the spinous processes. But there are few instances of this kind, and any physician can soon make himself familiar with what they are.

Symptoms that commence, or end, "deep in the chest," or "deep in the thoracic cavity," as the expression occurs in several instances, we have endeavored to represent by the arrow commencing, or terminating, as the case may be, in about the middle of the chest antero-posteriorly. Where the darting pains commence or terminate in the right scapula, we place the corresponding head or tail of the arrow upon the scapula, as near the point of origin or termination of the pain as the language indicates. And with all the symptoms which are given as terminating in the back, without any mention of the scapula as the place at which they stop, we have carried the arrows through below this bone, except Ambra grisea, because with so many of them, the shoulder-blades are so especially named for all symptoms that commence, or terminate at, or pass between them, that we infer that when the back, and not the scapulæ, is given, as the stopping place, a point between these bones must be meant. With Ambra grisea we had to place the arrow somewhat above the inferior angle of the scapula, in order to find room or a place for it. The plates must ultimately be given on a scale three or four times as large, then there will be ample room and all confusion will be avoided.

The dotted lines for the arrows across the scapula are to indicate that all such pains pass *between* this and its mate.

In some instances, we have had much difficulty in placing the arrows satisfactorily, from the fact that the language of the symptoms is so indefinite as to location. The expressions, "stitches from without inward," and "stitches from within outward in the right side of the chest," are common, without telling where, or at what point they occur, so we have had to infer the place, either from some facts in connection with other symptoms, or from some results we have known in practice. We do not claim these are all right, but thought best to give them, so as to insure future observation and make them right if they are wrong. In the majority of instances, however, the exact points of origin and termination are given, or near enough to this for all practical purposes; and every physician must feel a great satisfaction, or reliability, in this; while the defects we have named show more and more clearly, as we go on with this work, the great necessity there is for all provers, in the future, naming the exact locality, together with the direction and extent, where they have these latter qualities, of all the symptoms they experience.

The absence of Aconite from the previous plates, and also from the one now given, may seem singular to many, but we have to be governed by the recorded symptoms, in all instances where we have no facts outside of these. In the view of the left side this drug will have its place.

AMBRA GRISEA.

"Lancination in the chest extending to the back; in the right half of the chest a violent lancination arresting the breathing."

ARNICA.

1. "Dull stitches in the thoracic cavity through the sternum, from without inward." 2. "Cutting thrusts between the scapulæ, extending into the thoracic cavity, when walking." 3. "Stitch, at every inspiration, in the right side of the back, extending from the last ribs up to the axilla." 4. "Cramp like pain in the cervical vertebræ, accompanied by dull stitches from within outward."

ASAFŒTIDA.

"Stitches (lancinations, darting, etc.,) in the chest, in the right half of the chest, in the region of the right ribs, after a meal, with oppression; pinching pricking in the region of the right ribs; sticking with pressure in the right side or in the sternum, from within outward; also in the right thoracic cavity, or in the region of the right ribs toward the spine." The expression, "right ribs," we infer must here mean some point from the middle to the lower right ribs, thus according with the common expression "under" or "behind the ribs," the *lower* ribs being always understood.

BELLADONNA.

1. "Quickly passing lancinations under the last two ribs, as with a dull knife, by the side of the ensiform cartilage and above the false ribs." 2. "Fine stitches under the clavicle from before backward, during a walk." Though the side is not indicated by the language of either of these symptoms, we place the arrows both upon the right side, as Belladonna is so much more prominent in its action upon the right lung; but more especially have we done so with the latter symptom from the fact of recently obtaining so marked an effect from this drug in the 20,000th potency in *curing* a patient who had a cavity in the apex of the right lung from tuberculous ulceration, with an entire suspension of the menstrual function for nearly a year, and the pulse running at 130 and over per minute for a long time.

BERBERIS VULGARIS.

1. "Sticking pain, or sticking pain with pressure, more or less acute, frequently recurring and long continued, in one or the other lumbar region, at times in the region of the kidneys, at others, a little above or below, extending outward and forward in the side of the abdomen, or into the region of the hips, or into the dorsal spine or the small of the back, into the region of the bladder or the inguinal region, or extending from the region of the kidneys in a straight direction into the abdomen sometimes accompanied with a feeling of numbness, lameness, and as if bruised." All given with the plano-convex figure upon the arrow to indicate pressure with the sticking pain. 2. "Deep-seated, acute lancinating pain in the iliac bone of one or the other side, extending obliquely inward and downward toward the small of the back, sometimes accompanied with bubbling stitches darting into the part to a considerable depth." We locate the arrow for this according to the language "inward and downward," though it would be inward and a little *upward* to pass to the small of the back. 3. "Sudden stitch darting from the side of the neck into the upper arm." 4. "Lancinations from the lower region of the dorsal vertebræ through the chest, arresting the breathing." The arrow for this must necessarily pass upward and forward, to go "through the

chest" from the lower dorsal vertebræ, and so we have placed it.

BORAX VENETA.

1. Stitching or darting pain from without inward, through the upper portion of the right lung, posterior to the second rib. This is not from the Materia Medica, but is given as a result from a case in practice, which we will endeavor to give in detail under the head of "confirmations" by and by. 2. "Sudden stitches from within outward in the right side of chest, on lifting the arm." The location of this symptom not being given, we place the arrow in the upper part of the right chest, as the more probable locality, from the fact of the pain being excited by raising the arm. 3. "Fine prickings, extending from the back into the chest, in the evening," represented below the scapula, as this is not named in connection with the symptom. 4. "Tightness of the chest, with constrictive oppression of the breathing on going up stairs; he is then obliged to take a deep inspiration, which is always accompanied by an intensely-painful drawing stitch from without inward in the right side of the chest." 5. "Shortness of breath, after going up stairs, he cannot speak a word, and, when he speaks, he has a stitch from without inward in the right side of the chest; he experiences this same symptom when running, and when making a bodily effort which heats him." 6. "Arrest of breath when lying in bed; he has to jump up and catch breath; whenever he does this he experiences a cutting in the right side of the chest from without inward." 7. "Stitches between the ribs of the right side, so painful that he cannot lie on this side, with intensely painful drawing and sudden arrest of breath, which obliges him to snap for breath; when lying on the painful side the pain immediately arouses him from sleep." Though the exact locality of all these pains is not given, as will be seen, yet they are all essentially one symptom; at least the stitches are so similar, that we illustrate them with one hook and arrow, placed to correspond with results which we have seen from Borax upon acute pains in the chest, posterior to the right mamma.

BRYONIA.

1. "Pricking pain below the right nipple from within outward, in the cavity of the chest; these prickings are only felt during an inspiration." 2. "During an inspiration, stitch through the chest to the scapulæ." This is represented

as going through the chest just below the right mamma, as we have seen better effects from Bryonia upon acute pains in this part of the chest than any other.

CALCAREA CARBONICA.

"Violent stitches from the thoracic cavity, extending through the spinal column and coming out between the scapulæ."

CAMPHORA.

"Painful, drawing-stitches through and between the scapulæ, extending into the chest when moving the arms for two days."

CARBO VEGETABILIS.

1. "Violent dull stitches, like shocks from within outward, in the lower part of the right side of the chest." 2. "Deep stitch in the right side of the chest from without inward, when breathing deeply."

CASTOREUM.

"Painful sticking in the scapulæ, or between the shoulders, through the chest as far as the pit of the stomach, aggravated by inspiration."

CAUSTICUM.

"Stitches commencing deep in the chest and coming out at the back."

COCCULUS.

"Several stitches through the abdomen and the lower part of the back, from before backward, early in the morning, when in bed."

COLCHICUM.

"Lancinating tearing, deep in the right breast, through to the back."

DIGITALIS.

"Dull, clawing stitches along the lower border of the ribs, below the right axilla."

DULCAMARA.

1. "Dull stunning stitch in the chest below the right clav-

icle from without inward." 2. "Dull stitching pain in the right side of the chest, in the region of the third rib, especially when pressing on the part, when the pain went to the small of the back and extended between the shoulders; with stitches in one of the borders of the left scapula, during inspiration." 3. "Lancinating pain from the middle of the sternum to the dorsal spine when sitting, it goes off when rising." As this does not say "between the scapulæ" the common expression where the symptom ends there, we carry the arrow to the dorsal spine below the scapulæ.

GUAIACUM OFFICINALE.

"Continued stitches, finally terminating in one, close below the right scapula, they seem to come from the middle of the right half of the chest, and are increased by an inspiration."

HEPAR SULPHURIS.

"Stitching pain in the side of the chest, in the direction of the back."

INDIGO.

1. "Severe sharp stitch in the middle of the sternum, passing through the chest when sitting." 2. "Stitch in the region of the lower false ribs, toward the small of the back."

JUNCUS EFFUSUS.

"Stinging in the sternum or darting from the third false ribs as far as into the nipple."

KALI BICHROMICUM.

1. "Pain extending from the small of the back to the nape of the neck, and shooting through to the sternum, preventing him working for four weeks." 2. "Stabbing from third cervical to fifth dorsal vertebræ, striking forward through the chest to the sternum, increased on motion, with inability to straighten the spine after stooping; it prevented him from working for six weeks." 3. "Stitches under the sternum through to the back." Upon the arrow representing this symptom we have placed two tails, one just posterior to the sternum, the other under the right mamma. The reason for this will be found under the head " confirmations," on a subsequent page.

KALI CARBONICUM.

" Stinging pain as from blows and bruises, in the right scapula, when in motion; it may be felt as far as the chest."

KALI HYDRIODICUM.

" Pain as from soreness with sticking deep in the chest, in the region of the right lowermost rib, in the evening."

KALI NITRICUM.

" Sticking below the short ribs of the right side toward the back apparently behind the liver."

KREASOTUM.

" Stitch in the right side, arresting the breathing, sometimes, extending as far as under the scapula, and so violent that she imagines she will fall."

LACHESIS.

1. " Stitches, sometimes extending to the liver or kidneys," from the " small of the back " we are left to infer, from what immediately precedes and follows this symptom in the Symptomen Codex. 2. " Stitch in the lower part of the breast in front, from without inward." This does not say which side, but from the two preceding symptoms we infer it must be the right breast that is meant.

LACTUCA VIROSA.

" Stitches in the right chest, with subsequent sensation of spasmodic twitching, or in the lower part of the chest toward the back, in the region of the cartilages of the upper false ribs."

LAUROCERASUS.

1. " Stitches in the chest from the back to the sternum." 2. " Stitches in the sternum, also in the middle or in the lower part, also extending to the back, in the evening, during an inspiration."

MAGNESIA CARBONICA.

" Stitch in the small of the back, on the right side, from without inward, followed by jerking stitches in the small of the back."

MAGNESIA MURIATICA.

"Contraction of the chest, with oppressed breathing and dull stitches, from without inward, in the right side of the chest near the nipple, after supper."

MANGANUM.

"Violent stitches in the right half of the chest, near the sternum as if from without inward; nothing can relieve them."

MERCURIUS SOLUBILIS.

1. "Acute pain striking forward through the chest from the right scapula." This is given as the result of clinical experience by a brother practitioner in a distant city. 2. "When sneezing and coughing, between the acts of respiration, he feels a stitch in the anterior and superior portion of the chest, extending through to the back; the chest feels contracted and squeezed together by the stitch."

NICCOLUM.

"Stitch striking from the back to the pit of the stomach, in the afternoon when sitting."

NITRIC ACID.

"Violent stitch in the upper part of and within the right ribs, through the abdomen and back."

OLEUM ANIMALE.

"Violent stitch in the upper part of the right chest, near the sternum, as with a red-hot needle, the burning at that spot continuing a long time after."

PÆONIA.

"Throbbing through the right chest and extending posteriorly up to the nape of the neck, where the throbbing terminates in intermittent pinching." Figures of a heart are placed upon the line of this symptom to indicate throbbing.

PHELLANDRIUM.

"Violent stitch through the right mamma near the sternum, through to the back between the shoulders and then striking downward into the right side of the os sacrum, which is very painful on drawing breath, after dinner."

PHOSPHORUS.

1. "Stitches in the lumbar vertebræ, from without inward, extorting screams." 2. "Cutting from the middle of the sternum to the right scapula, worse during an inspiration, less during motion."

PULSATILLA.

"Sticking in the small of the back, afterward the pain extends into the abdomen, where it becomes cutting and sticking and arrests the breathing, followed by a creeping; heaviness and a drawing sensation in the head, accompanied with vanishing of sight and hearing, afterward dullness, as if he had cold water poured over him."

RAPHANUS SATIVUS.

"Pain in the chest, particularly when eating and coughing, less when drinking, the pain being of an aching and sticking character, extending from the pit of the stomach to the throat-pit and frequently to the back."

RATANHIA.

"Several dull stitches from the spine to the pit of the stomach."

RUTA.

"Painful darting in the dorsal spine, opposite the pit of the stomach; this becomes worse by pressing on the part, in which case a pain is felt under the last short ribs extending into the abdomen afterward and arresting the breathing."

SAMBUCUS.

"Sharp stitches from within outward, in the region of the right scapula, interiorly, most violent during rest."

SARSAPARILLA.

"Violent, continual drawing-stitches in the right cervical muscles, from the clavicle to the os hyoides."

SENEGA.

"Oppression of the chest, with slight shooting pains through the chest in the direction of the scapulæ, returning the first ten days at indefinite periods, especially in the open air and during a walk."

SEPIA.

"Stinging in the scapula, extending as far as the side and chest, only when sitting and walking fast; the stitching ceases when walking moderately, or when leaning against the affected side, mostly in the evening and afternoon."

SILICEA.

"Violent stitch through the right side of the chest. Stitch through to the back." These two, we take it, are really one symptom, so represent them with one arrow.

SPIGELIA.

"Dull sticking-pinching pain below the right nipple, in the thoracic cavity, from within outward, more violent during an inspiration."

SPONGIA.

"Violent prickings in the right side of the chest, from within outward."

STAPHYSAGRIA.

1. "Sharp stitches commencing in the posterior region of the right ribs, and winding round as far as the cartilages." 2. "Sharp stitches in the region of the fourth costal cartilage of the right and left side, at intervals of several seconds and lasting longer than usual; they press slowly from within outward, independent of breathing."

SULPHUR.

"Stitch from the right chest to the scapula."

TARAXACUM.

"Continuous dull stitch in the right scapula from within outward."

THUJA.

"Stitch in the back through the chest from below upward."

VALERIANA.

"Sudden stitches in the chest and in the region of the liver from within outward, causing him to start."

This completes the list of those drugs having acute pains of a darting or stitching character, which pass from point to point in the chest, or from this to other parts, in a manner that can be represented by a side view of the right side of the body. As was the case with the remedies illustrated heretofore, by a front view of the chest, the symptoms of each of those now given are all really different from those of any of the others, although the position of the arrows of some corresponds with that of others. Such symptoms, however, are similar in appearance only, not in fact. For instance, Bryonia and Phosphorus each have upon the plate now given an arrow extending from the front of the chest to the right scapula; but mark the difference: Phosphorus has the symptom, "Cutting from the middle of the sternum to the right scapula, worse during an inspiration, *less during motion;* and Bryonia has this: "During an inspiration, stitch through the chest to the scapulæ," the plural termination of this last word indicating of course, that the pain passes to both the right and the left scapula. Therefore to make this symptom complete in the illustration, it must be represented by another arrow upon the left side, extending through to the left scapula. Again the pain in this instance does not start from the middle of the sternum, as with Phosphorus, but from just below the mamma, according to our experience; besides, we all know that the acute pains of Bryonia are almost invariably greatly *aggravated*, not ameliorated, by motion, as is the case with the quoted symptom of the former drug.

And so it is with the other drugs represented on the plate by arrows similarly located, they are all really different, and there is nothing we would like more than to go through the comparisons of all that appear similar, as we did with several such in our last chapter, for if we mistake not, there is no field in the whole range of our science of therapeutics so rich in material for instruction as this. With those drugs whose arrows do not correspond in position, how strangely distinct they stand forth. Take for instance Dulcamara and Nitric acid. There are pains of each of these which start from near the same point in the upper part of the right chest, but with the former they shoot to between the shoulders and downward to the small of the back, while with the latter they descend into the abdomen and down "through the back." Then take Kali bichromicum, Phellandrium, Berberis, etc., how peculiarly strange their symptoms are, and how instructive to the true student of Homœopathy.

In order to make our illustrations complete, we have copied the symptoms given in this chapter from both the chest and back symptoms of the Materia Medica.

We will here mention what we had forgotten to speak of before, and that is, the absence of a representation of Arsenicum from the upper right lung, upon the plates thus far given, may seem like an omission, after what we already know of its action there. But the symptoms of this drug in that locality are more *fixed* acute pains than they are darting from point to point, and must be represented by another device than the arrow.

CHAPTER III.

PAINS OF LEFT SIDE.

In this chapter will be found a plate of the left side of the body, giving the darting or stitching pains of the chest and back to be represented by such a view. A different course has been pursued, in one respect, with illustrating symptoms in this, from that which was followed in either of the preceding chapters. For instance, we have only illustrated those darting pains which are definitely located by their language. At least the only exception to this is Causticum in its symptom, "stitches at night, without arresting the breathing, as if a knife were thrust into the left side of the chest in front, and in the back," etc. This being so distinct from all other drug stitches in the left chest, no other having anything at all like it, we thought it important that it should have a place, and if the position given its arrows is not exact, it can matter but little, as it must almost certainly be the remedy indicated for pains shooting at one and the same time, from before backward, and from the back forward into the left lung. It is certainly the only remedy yet recorded for such a combination. Aside from this, the acute pains of those drugs which are simply mentioned as extending through the left chest to the back, or of those from the latter into the chest, without either their origin or termination being given, we have not attempted to locate, because of the uncertainty.

It would have been better had this course been pursued from the first, and thus have avoided confusion, and made every pain represented a fixed and positive fact; but in new things like this it is impossible to attain perfection at once. Experience and reflection must be had to suggest improvements. The correction may be readily made upon the plates previously given, by running through the quoted symptoms, and finding those pains not positively located by the language, and then drawing a line of red ink through the abbreviated name of each drug on the illustrated page where there is any uncertainty about it. There are not more than one-fourth, we think, if there is that, which will be found in doubt, and then the balance will stand out clear and distinct as could be wished.

The stitching pains of uncertain location in the left chest we copy, and give at the close of the list of those that are definite. This is done to ensure observation that will properly locate them. They are clearly too important to be entirely overlooked, and this was our reason for endeavoring to represent all such, the best we could, in the front and right side views; but the course now adopted to secure them attention, but not an illustration until they are properly defined, is clearly much the best.

In comparing the results, after pursuing the course named, we find, too, much less similarity in position among the arrows representing the various drugs, on the present plate, from that of its predecessors. Indeed there is none of this whatever excepting beneath the left clavicle, and in the left præcordial region, and this leads us still more to think there is a possibility, at least, that had provers stated exactly the location, direction and extent of all the darting pains experienced by them, no two drugs would be found alike in this respect, that we should probably not have had to go beyond this one fact for a certainty in the remedy indicated, nor required a corroboration in other symptoms. But be this as it may, it will be seen in regard to the stitches beneath the clavicle, there is really no similarity between them, though in the representation there is so much of an appearance of this. Kali carbonicum, for instance, has: "Dull painful stitches in the chest, from without inward, under the left

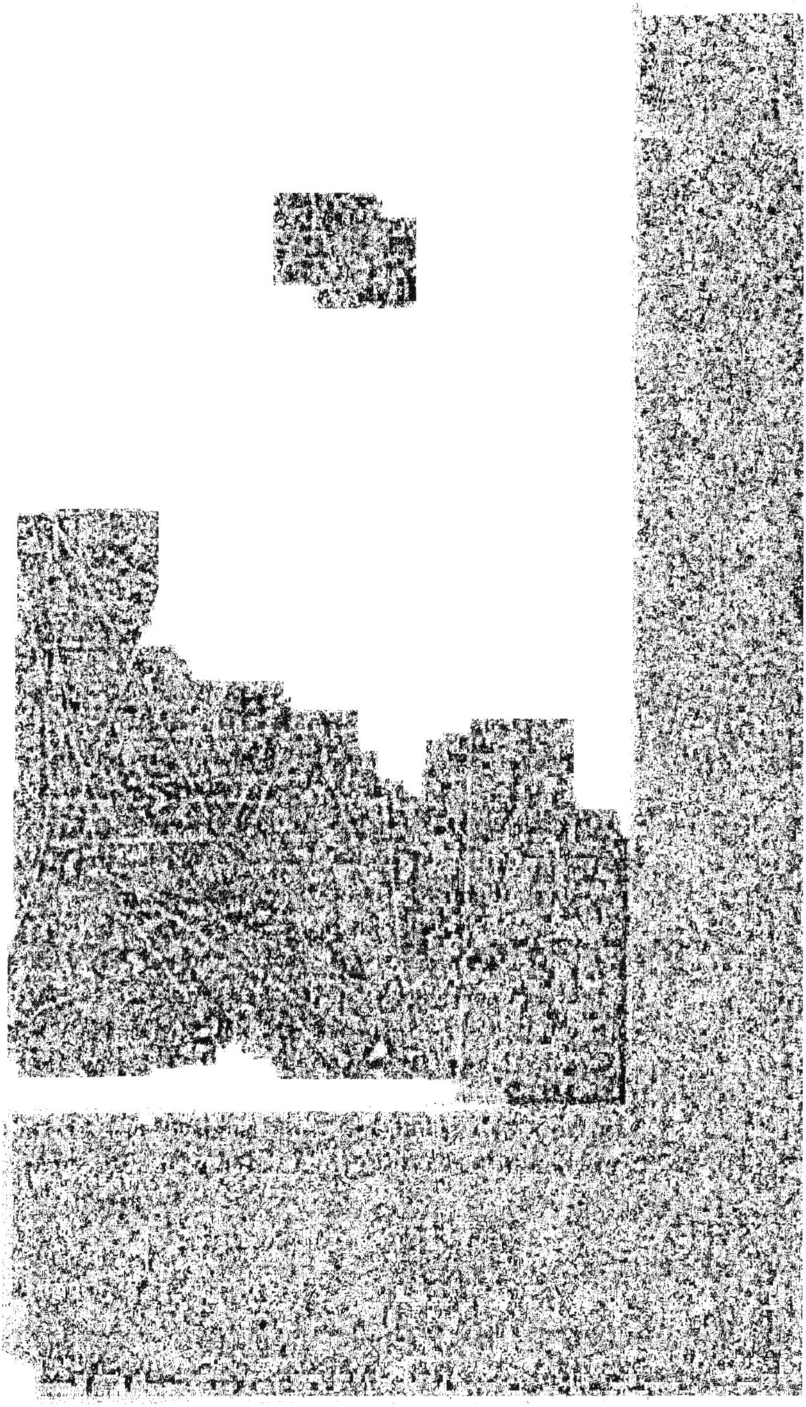

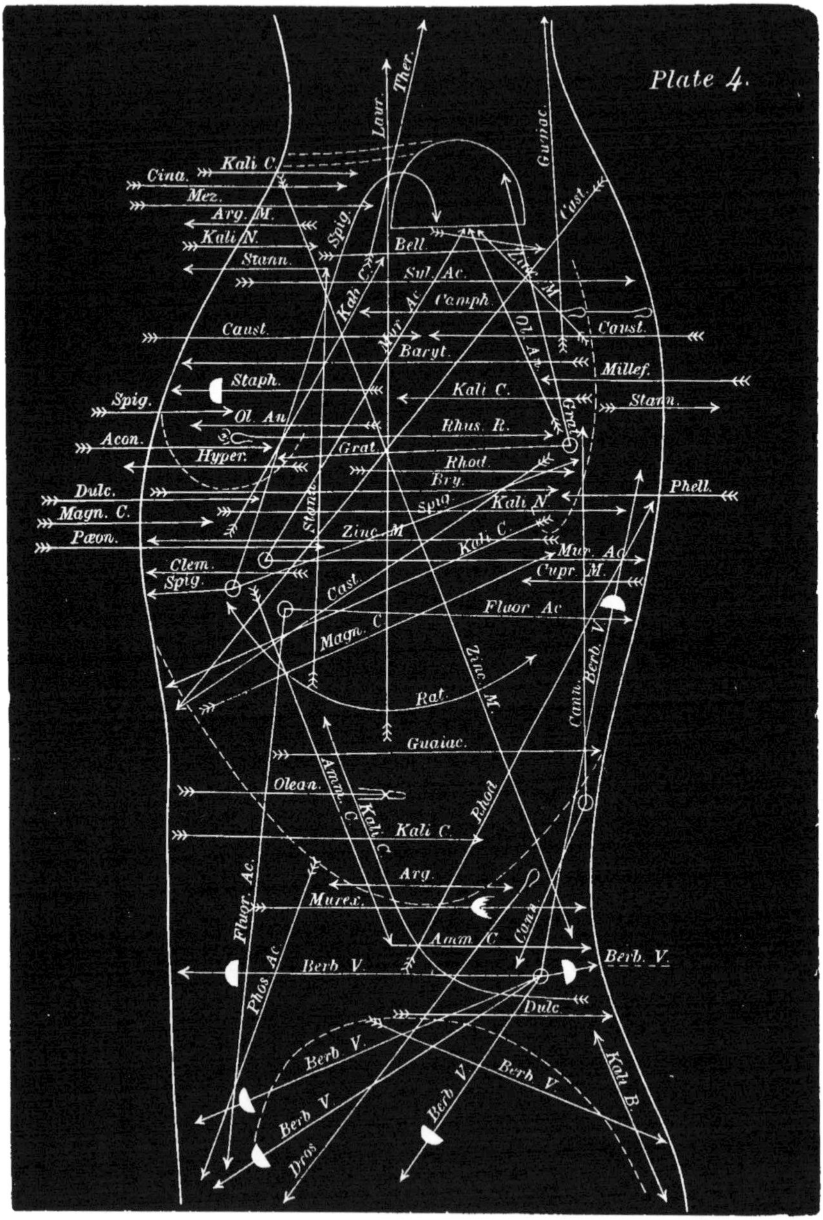
Ther.
Laur.
Guaiac.
Kali C.
Cina.
Mez.
Arg. M.
Kali N.
Stann.
Spig.
Bell.
Kali C.
Sul. Ac.
Cast.
Zinc. M
Camph.
Mur. Ac.
Ol. An.
Caust.
Caust.
Baryt.
Millef.
Staph.
Kali C.
Stann.
Spig.
Ol. An.
Rhus. R.
Grat.
Acon.
Hyper.
Grat.
Rhod.
Bry.
Phell.
Dulc.
Magn. C.
Spig.
Kali N.
Stann.
Pæon.
Zinc. M
Kali C.
Mur. Ac.
Clem.
Cupr. M.
Spig.
Cast.
Fluor. Ac.
Magn. C.
Berb. V.
Zinc. M.
Cann.
Rat.
Guaiac.
Olean.
Amm. C.
Kali C.
Rhod.
Kali C.
Arg.
Murex.
Fluor. Ac.
Amm. C
Cann.
Berb. V.
Berb. V.
Phos. Ac.
Dulc.
Berb. V.
Berb. V.
Berb. V.
Kali B.
Berb. V.
Dros.
Plate 4.

clavicle, *going off* for a short while by *pressing on the parts*, in the evening;" while Cina has: "*Two* dull, piercing stitches, in *quick succession*, near the sternum beneath the left clavicle, during a deep inspiration, he feels *much pain* when *pressing* on the part," making the two the *exact opposites*, in the fact that the same agency, namely pressing upon the part, relieves the one and aggravates the other. But this distinction would appear to be hardly required, for it will be seen that Kali carbonicum has five other arrows on the present plate, whereas Cina has but one. Again, Mezerum is markedly different from either of the foregoing, though it, too, has an arrow similarly placed beneath the left clavicle. Its symptom, however, leaves no doubt, as will be seen by quoting it in full: "Stitches in the left side of the chest, beneath the clavicle, *going and coming with the regularity of musical beats*, extending deep into the chest, shortly after, only a simple aching aggravated by inspiration, and returning for some days in succession." Of the other short arrow, belonging to Kali nitricum below those representing the preceding drugs, and extending from without inward, it is only necessary to say it simply extends through the upper part of the sternum.

While upon this point it appears important to call attention to the following under Dulcamara: "*Deep cutting pain* in the left side of chest, close below the clavicle, going off by pressing on the part." But whether this is a *fixed* deep cutting pain, or extends from one point to another, as the expression would seem to indicate, and if the latter, whether it passes antero-posteriorly, perpendicularly, or transversely, is so uncertain, we thought best not to represent it, but call attention to it in this manner, as it is too marked a symptom to pass by in silence. It will be seen that it is ameliorated by the same that the illustrated symptom of Kali carbonicum is in the same locality, namely, "by pressing on the part," but other symptoms will leave no doubt as to the one indicated.

Of the arrows in the præcordial region which correspond to each other in position, the same fact holds that does in the left infra-clavicular region. The symptoms of the drugs there represented are really so different, as will be seen by referring to them, and the concomitants so unlike, there can hardly be a mistake in regard to which remedy might be called for, if any care is taken in comparing them. Aside from these two localities, there are no two or more other arrows at all similarly located in the whole of this left side view. The nearest that any come to it are Zincum and Oleum animale, from the left scapula to the axilla, but the distinction is clear, as seen by the fact that the former has: "*Continuous* stitching in the *border* of the left scapula, toward the axilla;" and Oleum animale "a *few* pointed and painful stitches from the left scapula" not from its border "to the axilla." The apparent similitude between Bryonia and Kali nitricum is at once dispelled, when we reflect that the arrow belonging to the former on this plate is the mate to the one upon the right side going through to the right scapula. Besides, Kali nitricum does not go to the scapula but through the chest below the mamma, toward the back. In all the rest of this plate, as just stated, there is no resemblance whatever in the position of the arrows, when we consider their direction and the points between which they pass. Does not this fact, then, warrant as extravagant hopes, almost as could be raised of its great value, and is it not of the very highest importance both to Homœopathy and to suffering humanity that the illustration should be *fully* completed, for the whole system, as speedily as possible? But the labor required to do this is appalling.

All the darting pains passing through the *centre* of the chest antero-posteriorly, or the reverse, were illustrated in the last chapter, and are therefore not reproduced here.

ACONITUM.

Weight in the chest, accompanied with a number of fine but violent stitches in the left breast, from without inward.

AMMONIUM CARBONICUM.

Violent stitches in the left side of the chest, commencing in the præcordial region, and then moving downward toward the side, and afterward toward the back.

ARGENTUM METALLICUM.

1. Fine stitches in the upper part of the sternum from within outward. 2. Horizontal cutting, as with a knife, in the region of the left false ribs. 3. Lancination across the last rib of the left side when stooping sideways and leaning on the arm. As the last two are probably, one symptom, we so represent them on the plate.

BARYTA CARBONICA.

Dull stitches through the left scapula, coming out at the chest.

BELLADONNA.

Stitches shooting through the left axilla, and from a point on the front of the left chest, two or three inches to the right of the axilla, through to about the centre of the outer border of the left scapula. This is not hitherto a recorded symptom, but is from a case in practice which will be found in the chapter on "Confirmations."

BERBERIS VULGARIS.

1. Sticking pain, or sticking pain with pressure, more or less acute, frequently recurring and long continued, in one or the other lumbar region, at times in the region of the kidneys, at others a little above or below, extending outward and forward in the side of the abdomen, or into the region of the hips, or into the dorsal spine, or the small of the back into the region of the bladder or inguinal region or extending from the region of the kidneys, in a straight direction into the abdomen, sometimes accompanied with a feeling of numbness, lameness, and as if bruised. 2. Deep-seated, acute lancinating pain in the iliac bone of one or the other side, extending obliquely inward and downward toward the small of the back, sometimes accompanied with bubbling stitches darting into the part to a considerable depth.

BRYONIA.

During an inspiration, stitch through the chest to the scapulæ.

CAMPHORA.

Painful drawing stitches through and between the scapulæ, extending into the chest, when moving the arms, for two days.

CANNABIS SATIVA.

Violent aching and fine painful stinging, for fifty days in the vertebræ at the base of the chest, the pain sometimes darted toward the loins or the scapulæ.

CASTOREUM.

Painful sticking in the scapulæ or between the shoulders through the chest as far as the pit of the stomach, aggravated by inspirations.

CAUSTICUM.

Stitches at night, without arresting the breathing, as if a knife were thrust into the left side of the chest in front and in the back, with great anguish and uneasiness, which obliges him to toss about in his bed without being able to sleep.

CINA.

Two dull piercing stitches in quick succession, near the sternum, beneath the left clavicle, during a deep inspiration, he feels much pain when pressing on the part.

CLEMATIS ERECTA.

Sharp stitches in the region of the heart, from within outward.

CUPRUM METALLICUM.

Broad stitches as with a knife, under the scapula, on the left side near the spinal column, independent of breathing.

DROSERA.

Drawing stitches from the left loin into the penis.

DULCAMARA.

1. Pain in the left side of the chest, in the region of the fifth and sixth ribs, as if a blunt knife were thrust in. 2. Dull stitch from within outward in the left loin, close above the hips, at every inspiration.

FLUORIC ACID.

Pain from the left side of the chest to the groins, increased by deep inspiration, particularly in the groin and back, like a stitch.

GRATIOLA.

Darting from the left scapula to the shoulder and mamma.

GUAICUM OFFICINALE.

1. Stitches in the left side below the true ribs, rather toward the back. 2. Frequent and continued stitches on the left side of the nape of the neck, from the scapula to the occiput, when moving about, also when holding the head still.

HYPERICUM PERFOLIATUM.

Continual stitches from within outward, through the left breast and sternum, aggravated by motion.

KALI BICHROMICUM.

Cutting pain in the outer left side of the sacrum, shooting up and down.

KALI CARBONICUM.

1. Stitches under the left mamma, and sometimes ascending deep in the chest, also in the evening. 2. Dull stitches deep in the left chest under the short ribs. 3. Dull painful stitches in the chest from without inward, under the left clavicle, going off for a short while by pressing on the parts in the evening. 4. An occasional stitch from the small of the back, through the left side of the abdomen, toward the chest. 5. Stitch from the apex of the scapula to the pit of the stomach, during fatiguing labor. 6. Violent stinging pain as from a sprain in the left scapula, extending into the chest.

KALI NITRICUM.

1. Violent stitch in the upper part of the sternum, from without inward, on the left side. 2. Stitches in the left side of the chest, toward the back, and below the left mamma.

LACTUCA VIROSA.

Dull sticking from the left chest to the scapula.

LAUROCERASUS.

Stinging tension in the left side when lying on it, extending up to the neck in the morning.

MAGNESIA CARBONICA.

1. Stitch from without inward in the præcordial region. 2. A stitch into the left region of the ribs, coming out below the left scapula when standing.

MEZEREUM.

Stitches in the left side of the chest, beneath the clavicle, going and coming with the regularity of musical beats, extending deep into the chest, shortly after only a simple aching, aggravated by inspiration, and returning for some days in succession.

MILLEFOLIUM.

Violent fine stitch in the middle of the left scapula from without inward, during an inspiration.

MUREX PURPUREA.

Stinging and burning under the left short ribs, toward the spine.

MURIATIC ACID.

Stitches deep in the præcordial region extending as far as the axilla and back, with stitches in the thigh extending to the knee, when sitting, going off when rising in the evening.

OLEANDER.

Fine stitches in the left chest. Stabbings in the left chest as with a knife. Pinching stitch in the left chest, through the false ribs. Dull stitches in the left side of the chest when walking. Of these we can only definitely locate the "pinching stitch," but copy the others here as they occur in this close connection in the Materia Medica.

OLEUM ANIMALE.

1. Darting in the mamma, when standing, from behind forward. 2. A few pointed and painful stitches from the left scapula to the axilla.

PÆONIA.

Dull stitches in the chest from before backward, as if through the heart.

PHELLANDRIUM.

Stitch in the lower end of the left scapula, from without inward.

PHOSPHORIC ACID.

Dull stitch in the left side between the lowest rib and the pelvis, through the whole cavity of the abdomen, more violent during an inspiration.

RATANHIA.

Several fine stitches under the left breast, along the ribs.

RHODODENDRON.

1. Painful sticking in the left side below the ribs, the stitches extending in the direction of the dorsal vertebræ, during rest. 2. Sticking pain in the middle of the left chest. He feels the pain as far as scapulæ, and it is increased by motion.

RHUS RADICANS.

Drawing and stitching pain, extending from the left side of the chest near the nipple, through to the left scapula, aggravated by coughing, sneezing, yawning, etc.

SPIGELIA.

1. Lancinating pain commencing below the left nipple and extending into the region of the scapula and the upper arm, more violent during deep inspirations. 2. Dull oppressive sticking in the heart, between the region where the beats of the heart are felt and the scrobiculus cordis; the same sticking is felt in and above the scrobiculus cordis and the chest is oppressed. These symptoms are all represented by three arrows extending in the proper direction from one circle. 3. Sharp stitches above the left nipple from without inward, when sitting bent while writing, recurring at various periods; the stitches disappeared speedily when raising his chest.

STANNUM.

1. Sharp broad stitches in the spine, between the scapulæ, from within outward. 2. Frequent cuttings through the chest from below upward and in front in the region of the upper ribs from within outward, independent of breathing. As this is copied from the midst of symptoms given as in the

left side of the chest, we think it, also, must belong there, and so place it.

STAPHYSAGRIA.

Sharp stitches in the region of the fourth costal cartilage of the right and left side, at intervals of several seconds and lasting longer than usual; they press slowly from within outward, independent of breathing.

SULPHURIC ACID.

Sudden violent and piercing stitch in the upper part of the left chest, extending to the back.

THERIDION.

Violent stitches high up in the chest, through the left shoulder as far as the neck.

ZINCUM METALLICUM.

1. Stitch in the upper part of the sternum, extending into the left lumbar region, with dread of stooping, early in the morning. 2. Stitches under the left scapula, extending to the forepart of the left region of the chest. 3. Continuous stitching in the border of the left scapula toward the axilla, so violent that it caused her to start, with mounting of heat to the head.

STITCHING PAINS IN THE LEFT CHEST, WHICH ARE UNCERTAIN, EITHER AS TO LOCATION, DIRECTION, OR EXTENT.

ACONITUM.

Shooting stitches in the pectoralis major muscle, and in the intercostal muscle of the left side.

ASAFŒTIDA.

Boring stitches in the left side and left half of the chest, from within outward.

BORAX.

At every inspiration stitch into the left side of the chest, as with a knife.

BOVISTA.

Stitch in the left side, extending through to the back.

CROTON TIGLIUM.

Fullness and weariness of the two cavities of the chest, with stitches in the left cavity and toward the scapulæ.

DULCAMARA.

Deep cutting pain in the left side of the chest, close below the clavicle, going off by pressing on the part.

LYCOPODIUM.

Stitches in the left side of the chest, also during an inspiration, and extending to the back; they almost hinder breathing.

MAGNESIA MURIATICA.

Stitches deep in the left side of the chest, independent of breathing. Stitches in the left side of the chest, from without inward, with soreness when touching the parts.

MERCURIUS SOLUBILIS.

Stabbing pain in the left side under the short ribs, during every inspiration.

MEZEREUM.

1. Sticking pain from the left side of the back through the chest, during an inspiration. 2. Sudden sharp stitches in the evening, near the spinal marrow, through the chest, extending into the cartilages of the left ribs.

MURIATIC ACID.

Dull stitch in the left side of chest, from without inward, with cough in the evening.

NATRUM CARBONICUM.

Stitches in the back, sometimes as far as the left side of the chest, evening and night.

NICCOLUM.

Stitch in the left chest, also striking to the inmost part of the chest and arresting the breathing, or causing one to start, or when walking and worse on drawing breath.

NITRUM.

Stitches in the left side of the chest, toward the back.

PHELLANDRIUM.

Sticking deep in the left chest. Pointed stitches below the left mamma.

SENEGA.

Oppression of the chest, with slight shooting pains through the chest in the direction of the scapulæ, returning the first ten days at indefinite periods, especially in the open air and during a walk.

STANNUM.

A sudden long stitch in the left side of the chest, one hand's breadth below the axilla, causing one to start.

SULPHURIC ACID.

Fine stitches deep in the left side of the chest, from with out inward, with arrest of breathing.

TARAXICUM.

Sticking in the left side toward the back.

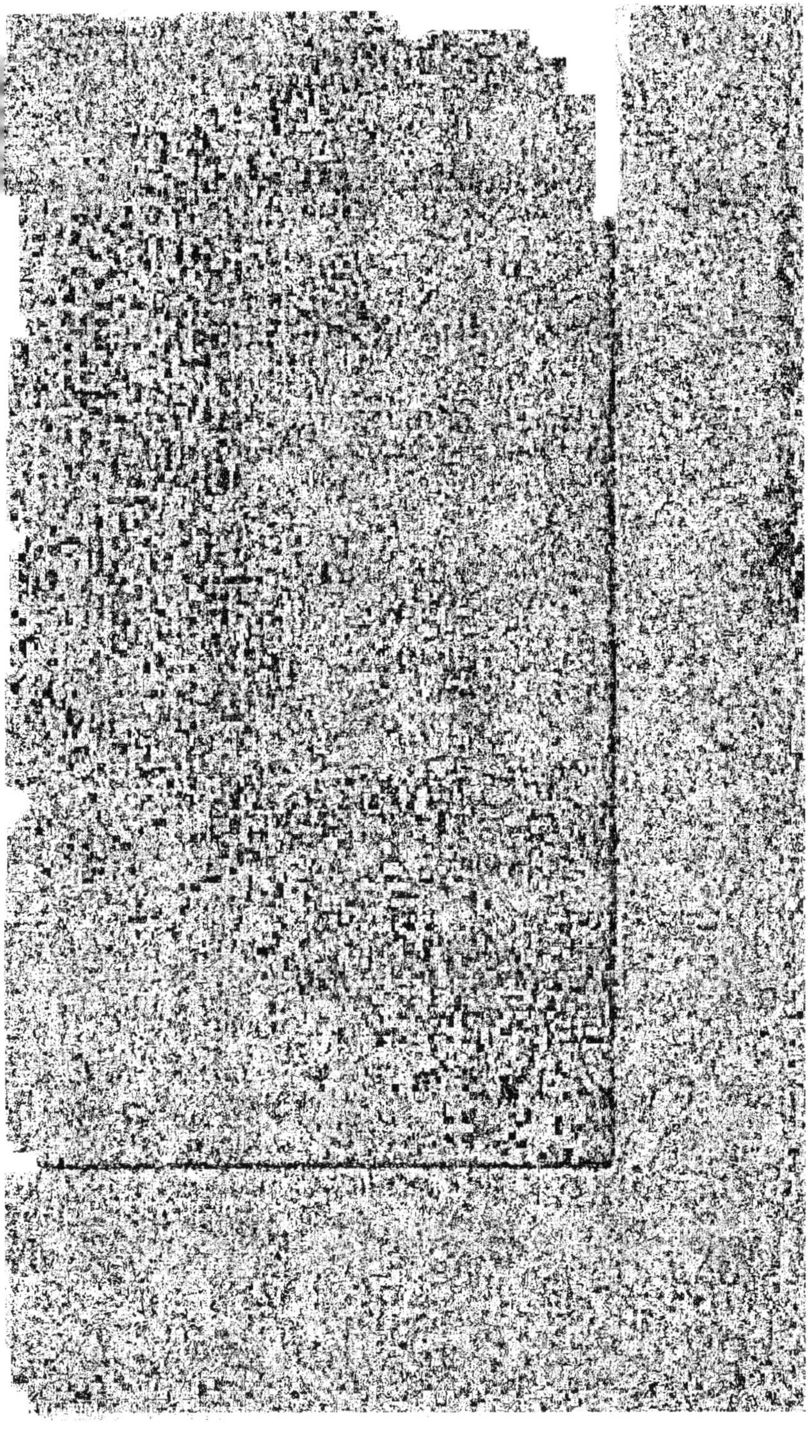

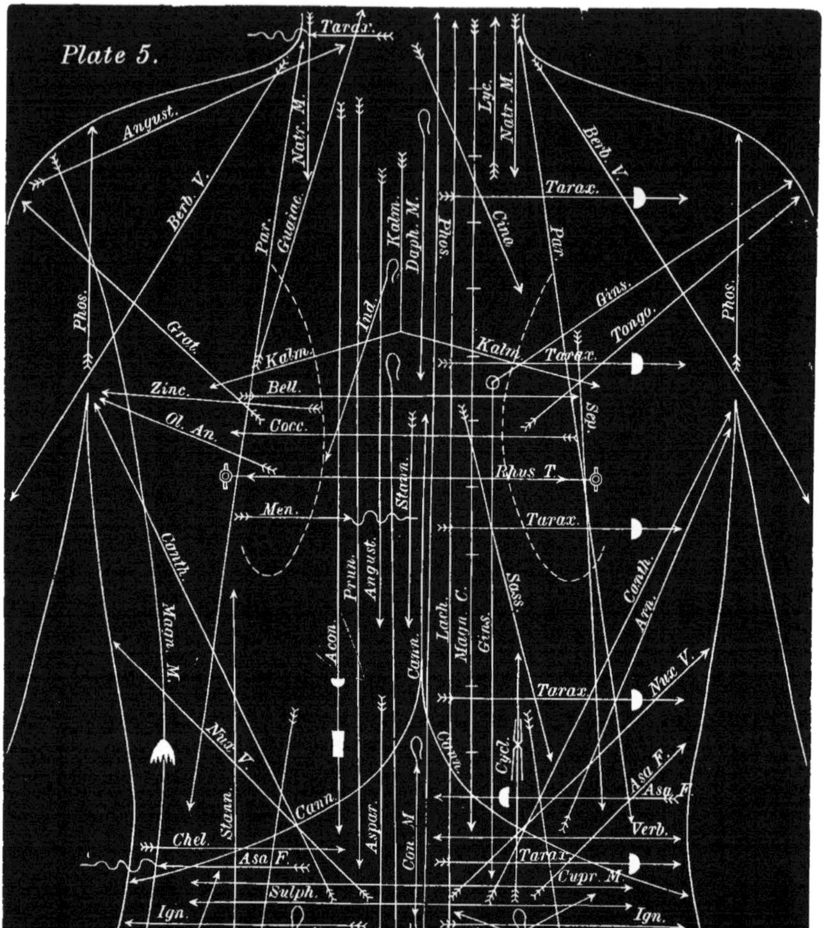

Plate 5.
Tarax.
Angust.
Natr. M.
Berb. V.
Lyc.
Natr. M.
Berb. V.
Tarax.
Par.
Guaiac.
Kalm.
Daph. M.
Phos.
Cina.
Par.
Phos.
Grot.
Ind.
Gins.
Tongo.
Phos.
Kalm.
Kalm.
Tarax.
Zinc.
Bell.
Sep.
Ol. An.
Cocc.
Rhus T.
Men.
Stann.
Tarax.
Canth.
Prun.
Angust.
Sass.
Magn. M.
Lach.
Magn. C.
Gins.
Canth.
Arn.
Acon.
Cann.
Tarax.
Nux V.
Nux V.
Cupr.
Cycl.
Asa F.
Asa F.
Stann.
Cann.
Verb.
Chel.
Aspar.
Con. M.
Tarax.
Asa F.
Cupr. M.
Sulph.
Ign.
Ign.
Natr. M.
Berb. V.
Magn. M.
Dros.
Dros.
Ferr. A.
Berb. V.
Ferr. A.
Alu.
Alu.
Alu.
Natr. C.
Asa F.
Phos.
Carb. A.
Zinc.
Kali B.
Dulc.
Ox. Ac.
Ox. Ac.
Dulc.
Kali B.
Zinc.
Carb. A.
Hep.
Kali B.
Hep.

CHAPTER IV.

PAINS IN THE BACK.

In this chapter we complete the illustrations of the darting pains in the chest, by giving a view of those in the back, but as no proper division can be made in these, with reference to the chest alone, the whole length of the back is given, and the corresponding pains for all parts thereof.

It will be seen that there are three new characters upon this plate not before used. Their explanation is as follows: The figure of a miniature *spade* signifies a *digging* pain; or, when placed upon an arrow, as in this instance, to illustrate a symptom of Aconite, extending down the left side of the spine, it is to represent a digging in connection with the "sticking" pain. The figure of the *cork-screw* is to illustrate a *boring* pain; with the arrow, a boring stitch. And the *ring*, with a short bar through it, upon either scapula, to illustrate a symptom of Rhus toxicodendron, stands for a sensation of *tension*, or a "tensive stitch," as it is there used.

Again we must call attention to the strange and unexpected distinctness given to drug symptoms by this method, where, before, nearly all appeared so similar, and because of this, so greatly confused. Among all the drugs illustrated upon this plate, no two are alike, even in the one symptom represented, excepting Cuprum, Sulphur, and Natrum muriaticum in their transverse stitches through the small of the back; but no one ought to make a mistake as to which of these remedies might be called for by such stitches, if they compare their other symptoms. In all else, where there is a similarity in the location, direction and extent of the arrows, the symptoms are so in the representation only, for by comparing the language upon which the illustrations are made, we in no instance have to go beyond the one symptom quoted of each, to establish which drug would be indicated.

Let us take those with arrows extending from the small of the back downward on to the thighs, for comparison. Oxalic acid has: "Acute pain in the *back*," not from the small of back, "*gradually* extending down to the *thighs*, occasioning ere long great torture." Dulcamara has: "*Drawing* from the small of the back *through* the thighs, *during rest*, with stitches in the part." Kali bichromicum: "Sharp shooting pains, *first* in the left, *afterward* in the right renal region, extending down the thigh, *aggravated by motion*." Zincum metallicum: "Violent *cutting* in the small of the back at the *least* motion, extending into the *calves* and *feet*, he is neither able to walk, stand, or lie down." Carbo animalis: "Stitch in the small of the back descending *along* the thighs, on *every inspiration*." While Hepar sulphur has: "Sharp *pressure*" "in the small of the back and the lumbar vertebræ, especially in the region of the sacro-iliac symphysis, extending into the *lower limbs*." So in all this there are no two alike, or even similar in their essential features.

Passing up the spine the same fact holds in a still more marked degree, for there is here but little similarity, in any respect, and this is more astonishing than all else, when we consider the important functions and the great length of the spinal cord. The only drugs that at all approach even an apparent resemblance in the illustrations, are Lachesis and Phosphorus, in their arrows ascending the spine; but how great the distinction between them; for the former has: "Stitches in the upper part of the back, or along the back from below upward, or in the whole back and in the nape of the neck, with stinging in the *right* arm and sensation as if it had gone to sleep, with *itching* on the *arms*, *hips*, and *lower limbs*." With Phosphorus, on the contrary, the arrow is to illustrate a "Darting pain, *during stool*, from the *os coccygis* through the spine *as far as the vertex*, the head being drawn backward by it." Stapysagria has: "Severe stitches along the *back*, from below upward," but the locality and extent are, of course, so uncertain from this language, that we have not attempted to illustrate it. It is not probably along the *spine*, or this would have been specially mentioned as in other instances.

Of those *descending* the spine, Aconite has: "Violent, sticking, *digging* pain," down the left side of the spinal column to the small of the back. Prunus spinosa: "Stitch from between the shoulders to the lumbar vertebræ on drawing deep a breath." Natrum carbonicum: "Rigidity and drawing between the scapulæ, in the open air," descending to the anus, where it terminates in a stitch when sitting or lying. And Magnesia carbonicum: "Violent tearing and darting," descending gradually from the neck along the back. Thus, it will be seen, that no two of these are alike, nor indeed at all similar in the character of the pain, though the direction and extent of the arrows of some of them correspond with that of others; and by this comparison it will also be seen, that Prunus is the *only* known remedy for a simple uncomplicated stitch descending the spine the greater portion of its length. Angustura has: "An incisive cutting from above downward in the dorsal spine," accompanied by the *same* descending *the sternum.* Stannum: "Slow intermittent dull stitches between the scapulæ toward the middle of the spine." Asparagus: "Sensation when sitting, as if something were darting through the small of the back toward the sacral vertebræ." And Ginseng: "Lancinations between the scapulæ, extending to the right shoulder, or along the spine down to the small of the back," etc.

Well, then, could anything be desired more clear in the distinctions, than is here displayed, where there would appear by simply reading, unaided by illustrations, such similarity and complication? In all the rest of this plate there is not the slightest resemblance in anything as regards the positions and directions of the arrows; while there are some most remarkable contrasts. See, for instance, the arrows representing Cantharis and Cannabis, two drugs so frequently called to mind in connection with diseases of the urinary organs.

There is one remaining point to which we will call attention, as showing the great practical value of this work. The fact that more or less severe pains, of some kind, so commonly occur in parts or organs before diseased action, whether acute or chronic, become, really seated in them, cannot have escaped the attention of every observing physician. Here, then, is the cry of distress and the call for relief before the part has become dangerously, often, indeed, before it has become even seriously involved; and, because of this, such pains must have been intended as the surest guides to the proper curative agent, that all cases might be reached before danger arises. In the very large majority of instances where the illustrations have shown but *one* remedy for a given pain, no other can be indicated but that, for such pain. Then, if all the pains of every drug were illustrated in their characteristic localities, direction, and extent, so that the physician could apply at once, the exact curative remedy pointed out by such symptoms, how grand would his successes and his mission be.

ACONITUM.

Violent sticking, digging pain, all along the spine, on the left side, down to the small of the back, aggravated by an inspiration.

ALUMINA.

Stitches in the left hip, extending to the small of the back, and to the loins; when taking an inspiration, the stitches come on again.

ANGUSTURA.

1. Dull stitches between the top of the left shoulder and the neck. 2. Pressure across the whole right side of chest and abdomen, as if these parts were compressed in front and behind, accompanied by an incisive cutting from above downward, in the sternum and in the dorsal spine, increased by inspiration and every movement of the trunk.

ARNICA.

Stitch, at every inspiration, in the right side of the back, extending from the last ribs up to the axilla.

ASAFŒTIDA.

1. Stitches in the region of the sacrum, extending down to the anus. 2. Boring sticking, in the left loin from within outward, going off during an inspiration. 3. Lancinations from the right loin toward the ribs? 4. Sticking, with pressure in the region of the right ribs toward the spine.

ASPARAGUS.

Sensation, when sitting, as if something were darting through the small of the back toward the sacral vertebræ.

BELLADONNA.

Repeated stitches, as if caused by the electric fluid, from the left scapula to the right.

BERBERIS VULGARIS.

1. Sudden stitch darting from the side of the neck into the upper arm. 2. Deep seated, acute lancinating pain in the iliac bone of one or the other side, extending obliquely inward and downward toward the small of the back, sometimes accompanied with bubbling stitches darting into the part to a considerable depth.

CANNABIS.

In the evening, when in bed, she feels a few dull stitches in both sides of the abdomen, the pain then darting upward along the back, terminating in stitches between the scapulæ, and afterward returning to the sides of the abdomen.

CANTHARIS.

Cutting in the region of the kidneys, extending to the axillæ.

CARBO ANIMALIS.

Stitch in the small of the back, descending along the thighs, on every inspiration.

CHELIDONIUM.

Dull stitches in the left loin, in quick succession, toward the back.

CINA.

Lancinating pain in the upper part of the spinal column toward the right scapula.

COCCULUS.

Stitches in the scapulæ from the right to the left.

CONIUM MACULATUM.

Stitches in the small of the back, with drawing through the lumbar vertebræ when standing.

CUPRUM METALLICUM.

Lancination in the small of the back in a transverse diree-tion.

CYCLAMEN EUROPEUM.

Piercing, pinching, dull stitches, recurring at equal periods of some seconds, on the right side of the spinal column (between the os innominatum and the last false rib), in the region of the kidney, more violent during an inspiration, which is interrupted by the extreme pain.

DAPHNE MEZEREUM.

Dull drawing stitches downward, between the shoulders, less when moving the parts.

DROSERA.

Lancinating tearing from the spinal marrow to the os ilium, when sitting.

DULCAMARA.

Drawing from the small of the back through the thighs, during rest, with stitches in the part, during motion, which are relieved by pressure.

FERRUM ACETICUM.

Stitch-like jerks, in the small of the back when walking, extending toward the hips rather than the upper parts;

more painful after sitting, or standing (almost as after straining the parts by lifting.)

GINSENG.

Lancinations between the scapulæ, extending to the right shoulder, or along the spine down to the small of the back, particularly on raising the trunk from a stooping posture, attended with oppression of breathing.

GRATIOLA.

Darting from the left scapula to the shoulder and mamma.

GUAIACUM OFFICINALE.

Frequent and continued stitches on the left side of the nape of the neck, from the scapula to the occiput, when moving about; also, when holding the head still.

HEPAR SULPHURIS.

Sharp pressure and pain, as from bruises; in the small of the back and the lumbar vertebræ, especially in the region of the sacro-iliac symphysis, extending into the lower limbs; the pain is felt when sitting, standing, or lying, and causes a sort of limping when walking.

IGNATIA.

Lancinations from the small of the back through the loins.

INDIGO.

Drawing lancinating pains, following the course of the left rhomboideus muscle.

KALI BICHROMICUM.

1. Cutting pain in the outer left side of the sacrum, shooting up and down. 2. Sharp shooting pains, first in the left, afterward in the right renal region, extending down the thigh, aggravated by motion.

KALMIA LATIFOLIA.

Sharp pain in the three superior dorsal vertebræ, extending through the shoulder blades.

LACHESIS.

Stitches in the upper part of the back, or along the back

from below, upward, or in the whole back and in the nape of the neck, with stinging in the right arm and sensation as if it had gone to sleep, with itching on the arms, hips, and lower limbs.

LYCOPODIUM.

Darting in the right cervical muscles from below upward.

MAGNESIA CARBONICA.

Violent tearing and darting in the nape of the neck, gradually descending along the back, and then passing off.

MAGNESIA MURIATICA.

1. A stitch into the right ilium toward the small of the back. 2. Stitches and burning in the region of the left shoulder down to the hip.

MENYANTHES TRIFOLIATA.

Dull boring stitching in the region of the left scapula, extending toward the spine.

NATRUM CARBONICUM.

Rigidity and drawing between the scapulæ, in the open air; or in the back, extending as far as the anus, in paroxysms, and terminating in a stitch when sitting or lying.

NATRUM MURIATICUM.

1. Sharp stitches transversely through the small of the back, close above the hips. 2. Stitches in the outer parts of the neck, from above downward, even in the night.

NUX VOMICA.

An illness in the afternoon, with violent stitching in the small of the back; afterward extending into the sides, and oppressing the breathing.

OLEUM ANIMALE.

A few pointed and painful stitches from the left scapula to the axilla.

OXALIC ACID.

Acute pain in the back, gradually extending down to the

thighs, occasioning ere long great torture, and continuing almost to the moment of death.

PARIS QUADRIFOLIA.

Stitches through the back, on either side of the back and nape of the neck.

PHOSPHORUS.

1. Stitches in the axillæ through the shoulders. 2. Darting pain, during stool, from the os coccygis through the spine, as far as the vertex, the head being drawn backward by it.

PRUNUS SPINOSA.

Stitch from between the shoulders to the lumbar vertebræ on drawing deep breath, arresting the breathing.

RHUS TOXICODENDRON.

Tensive cutting across the scapulæ.

SARSAPARILLA.

Stitches, sometimes lancinations near the spinal column, from the right scapula to the last false rib, increased during an inspiration, and arresting the breathing when taking deep breath.

SEPIA.

Stinging pain from the scapula down through the ribs, on the right side of the back, at every inspiration, lasting as long as this does, in every position of the body, but less when walking in the open air.

STANNUM.

1. Lancination in the left side of the back, from below upward, when standing. 2. Slow, intermittent, dull stitches, between the scapulæ, toward the middle of the spine.

SULPHUR.

Stitches transversely across the small of the back.

TARAXACUM.

1. Sharp boring stitches in the left side of the neck, from within outward. 2. Sticking pain with pressure in the whole spine toward the right side when lying, with difficult breathing, especially violent in the small of the back.

TONGO.

Stitch from the right scapula, through the shoulder, early in the morning.

VERBASCUM.

Cutting between the right loin and spinal column.

ZINCUM METALLICUM.

1. Continuous stitching in the border of the left scapula, toward the axilla, so violent that it caused her to start, with rising of heat to the head. 2. Violent cutting in the small of the back at the least motion, extending into the calves and feet; he is neither able to walk, stand, nor lie down.

STITCHING PAINS IN THE BACK WHICH ARE UNCERTAIN EITHER AS TO LOCATION, DIRECTION, OR EXTENT.

ALUMINA.

Fine stitches extending from the back to the ribs.

CHINA.

Sticking drawing toward the lumbar vertebræ.

DULCAMARA.

Dull stitches in both loins, with sensation as of squeezing from within outward, at every inspiration, while sitting bent (after a short walk).

HEPAR SULPHURIS.

Sticking pain in the side of the chest, in the direction of the back.

LAUROCERASUS.

Sticking, particularly on the right side, or toward the left shoulder.

LYCOPODIUM.

1. Stitches in the back, toward the small of the back, when sitting. 2. Sticking pain in the back, extending to the right scapula.

MORPHIUM ACETICUM.

Inspiration accompanied by sharp pain in the abdomen and along the spine.

SAMBUCUS.

Cutting pinching in the region of the last false ribs, toward the dorsal spine.

STAPHYSAGRIA.

Severe stitches along the back, from below upward. As this says along the *back*, not along the spine, it is, of course, uncertain as to the exact locality meant.

OMISSIONS.

The following symptoms were overlooked. They should have been illustrated in the side views.

ACONITUM.

Cutting pain extending in a circle from the spine to the abdomen, over the left hip. This is the only drug symptom of the kind, and should have been represented in the view of the left side.

ANGUSTURA.

The symptom of this remedy, illustrated on plate 1, by an arrow descending the sternum, and on the present plate by one descending the dorsal spine, would have been better given upon one of the side views, so as to have shown the natural connection existing between the acute pains in the two localities.

CALCAREA CARBONICA.

Spasmodic shooting pain from the small of the back toward the rectum.

KALI BICHROMICUM.

Cough causes pain in the middle of the sternum, darting through to between the shoulders.

KREASOTUM.

Sticking, with pressure through the whole chest, extending to the inner border of the scapula. To which scapula is uncertain, though it is probably to the right one, as most of the acute pulmonary pains of this drug occur in the right chest.

Chapter V.

CONFIRMATIONS.

Under this head we give cases from practice, which serve to confirm the symptoms of the various drugs as represented upon the plates. And to make this work general, and therefore so much more reliable than could be the case from the observations of two or three physicians, we ask our readers to forward us the results of their clinical experience in this direction, that such may be given in subsequent editions for the benefit of all. But to ensure the greatest reliability in this matter, we should ourselves very much prefer, and have no doubt others would desire, those cases which are cured by a single dose, or at most a very few doses of the high potencies, given at long intervals. Then we can all know that they are really *cures*, or that the medicine acted in a curative manner, and not in suppressing the symptoms to be followed by worse conditions. Again, it would be preferable to have those cases in which a long line of complicated chronic symptoms were broken up by the single dose—the key to the remedy being furnished by the position and direction of the arrows.

NATRUM MURIATICUM.

Dr. G. F. Foote has confirmed the symptom of this drug represented in Chapter I. by an arrow extending from the upper portion of the left lung, out into the left shoulder joint. The case was as follows: A lady aged about thirty years, had complained of this symptom some two years.

It was at times very severe and attended with many other symptoms which we cannot now give. She had, for some years previous to the appearance of the pain in the superior portion of the left lung, suffered greatly from facial neuralgia, upon the left side. But this was finally suppressed by local and other wrong treatment, and soon after, the disease seated in the lung. And as we have said she suffered from this some two years until Dr. F. took charge of the case. Upon ascertaining the locality and direction of the pain, he consulted the plates and found Natrum muriaticum to be the *only* remedy for such a symptom. Then by using this as a key to the case, he examined the Symptomen-Codex and there found, under this drug, all the symptoms of which his patient complained. Upon this he at once administered one dose of Natrum muriaticum 40,000. He said this entirely relieved all the suffering in the lung, in forty-eight hours time, when the facial neuralgia returned with great severity, and upon the same side as formerly, that is, the left side of the face. This continued very severe a few days, then gradually disappeared, without further medication, and the lady left here for the west some weeks after, averring that she was entirely cured of all the symptoms from which she had suffered so long and so much.

KALI BICHROMICUM.

In January we were called to a lady, aged some thirty-six years, who was suffering from chronic disease, the result of an attack of cholera morbus during the preceding August, and its partial suppression by a long course of Allopathic treatment. We say partial suppression for the reason that she was a long time in getting any relief, and was finally left with a chronic diarrhœa which troubled her daily. The evacuations generally occurred in the morning and forenoon, seldom in the afternoon or at night. She was much exhausted from it, and failing to get better by the treatment she had been pursuing, she went to a water cure establishment in November, and remained there some two months under treatment. This afforded some, though not entire relief to the bowels, but at the expense of driving so much of her disease to the lungs. At least she returned with a cough and other symptoms showing that a good deal of irritation was arising in the respiratory organs. We prescribed in succession Arsenicum, Phosphorus and Nux vomica in the order named, giving each several days to develop its action. but the results were not satisfactory. They ameliorated the cough and relieved the other chest symptoms somewhat, and as they did this the diarrhœa became worse, still they did not seem to us to act in a really curative manner. Under the latter named drug, however, there came a decided change of symptoms, for one day as we called, our patient was complaining that she was taken early that morning with very acute pains in the chest. Upon enquiry for their locality she said they darted through the right lung, from just below the right mamma, to the back below the right scapula. She also said that at the same time she suffered with very acute pains darting from just behind the left hip joint down on the outside of the left thigh, and sometimes to the calf of the leg; and that with all the rest she had severe acute pains about the left eye and left side of the forehead, from which she had suffered at times, very much, for years.

Not remembering the remedy for this combination of symptoms, we returned to our office and consulted our plates. These directed us to Kali bichromicum, and upon consulting the symptoms of this drug, in the Symptomen-Codex, we found the following: "Stitches under the sternum through to the back," and "Dull heavy pain in the right side of the chest, passing through to the back, recurring at intervals of twenty minutes, and lasting about that time." Then again: "Pain in the course of the left sciatic nerve, extending from behind the great trochanter to the calf of the leg, and "Darting pain down the outside of the left thigh. For the pain about the left eye and forehead we found the following: "Violent shooting pains from the root of the nose along the left orbital arch to the external angle of the eye," which "begins in the morning and increases till noon." Also this: "Soon after rising in the morning, darting pain in a small spot over the left eye, spreading over the forehead, but still remaining worse at the original spot; worse on motion; with gastric derangement, lasted several days." The lady always had gastric derangement with these headaches, and this attack commenced in the morning. We consequently prescribed Kali bichromicum 200, one dose, followed by Saccharum lactis, which in a day or two entirely relieved all the pains, and in a week so far relieved the diarrhœæ and recruited her strength, that she went down two flights of stairs, to her meals, a thing she had not before done since her first attack in August last. And she was able to go out to ride in two or three weeks, and now appears as well as ever.

Could science in any of its departments, go further, or be more exact than it was in this instance, in pointing out by the three different localities, the curative remedy for the case? True, the chest symptoms were not so exactly covered by the language of these, which we have quoted from the provings, as were the thigh and eye symptoms, but this was no doubt owing to those symptoms not having been carefully located by the provers. A re-proving would no doubt show pains in the chest to exactly correspond to the clinical result in this case. And we place the arrow to correspond with such result, but put two tails upon it, one to represent an acute pain passing from behind the sternum through to the back, according to the Materia Medica, and the other under the right mamma, upon the same arrow, to correspond with the facts of this cure.

BELLADONNA.

The symptom of this remedy, illustrated just beneath the left axilla, upon the plate given in Chapter IV., we have confirmed in the following case: September 15, 1869, we were called to a married lady, aged thirty years, who was suffering from a severe cough and pain in the chest. Upon inquiry the cough was found to be dry, harsh, rather hoarse, and somewhat hollow in sound, unattended by expectoration at any time, troublesome at nearly all hours during the day and evening, but worse in the afternoon from 3 P. M. to 5

P. M. There was hectic fever attending the other symptoms, with burning of the palms of the hands and soles of the feet, and an aggravation or rise of fever every day at 3 P. M., lasting two or three hours. Soreness of the throat, that is, a dry, raw, or smarting soreness was much complained of, and upon examination the whole mucous lining of the fauces was seen to present many resemblances to an acute inflammation thereof, though there was no swelling of the tonsils or other parts. All these symptoms had been of about six weeks' duration, and soon after they had set in there had arisen an acute pain in the left axilla, and in the front of the left lung at a point about three inches to the right of the axilla, which extended from both of these places backward through the lung to about the center of the outer border of the left scapula. This pain had been of three or four weeks' duration, and was gradually increasing in severity, though but little if any congestion had arisen in that or any other part of either lung, and we think the lungs were not yet really tuberculized, though they were certainly rapidly approaching, if not already upon the verge of this condition. The patient was much emaciated, weighing only ninety-seven pounds, though rather above the medium height. She was also much reduced in strength, being unable to take any out-door exercise, and had but little appetite. Pulse 110 to 120 per minute. Cough always excited by tickling in the throat.

To give still further evidence of the awful curse being daily inflicted upon mankind by the local treatment of disease, we will state that this condition and all these symptoms, followed soon after the suppression by topical application, of a chronic *leucorrhœa* and uterine irritation, from which the lady had suffered for some three or four years. She was at three different times, in the course of two years, subjected to treatment by cauterization and injections of Nitrate of Silver, twice and three times a week, for four or five months each time, causing much suffering that she would not fully recover from one of these assaults upon life till the next was made. The last of these periods was through the spring of 1869, and terminated but a few weeks before she was seized with the throat and lung disease described, and only just before the appearance of the latter did the female disease disappear.

The character of the cough and the symptoms of the throat were all so decided in calling for Belladonna that we prescribed this remedy in the 2000th potency, and awaited results, believing that it must control the acute pain promptly, because of its being so markedly indicated by the other symptoms. And the results were all that could have been desired. The pain and fever were among the first symptoms to yield, while the case progressed satisfactorily in all other respects, for three or four months, when the cough and irritation of the throat wholly subsided, and then the leucorrhœa and uterine irritation *reappeared just as they were before their suppression*, some five or six months previously. She said the identical pains and all other abnormal sensations in the genital organs returned, and were an exact repetition of their former action. We still allowed Belladonna to continue its work upon these as upon the throat and lung symptoms, and repeated it only once, to restore her, in two or three months longer, to such a state of health as she had not enjoyed during the preceding six or eight years.

CALCAREA CARBONICA.

We have confirmed the darting pains of this drug, illustrated by three arrows on plate 1, namely, by one arrow extending from the left into the right lung, across the center of the chest, and by two others, one from either lung, shooting up into the throat. The case was that of a married lady some thirty-one or two years of age, suffering from most inveterate symptoms of secondary syphilis. The disease was communicated to her some six or seven years since, through no fault of her own, and then suppressed by local treatment, only to be followed by constant suffering ever since. For three or four years she has discharged pus more or less freely from the rectum, and for the last two years has discharged large quantities of it almost daily, and latterly much blood also. She has in addition, been markedly dropsical for two or three years, principally of the nature of anasarca and ascites, and has been a victim to the worst form of constipation we have ever known. She asserts most positively that, in the last two years she has been no less than three or four different times, as long as four weeks at a time, or from one menstrual period to the next, without the slightest particle of fecal matter passing her bowels, and then they would work off in a diarrhœa, for a day or two, but after this resume the old condition, and go two, three, and sometimes the four weeks before another fecal evacuation; but would daily have discharges of pure pus, during all the intervening period. Well, after treating her at intervals, for a year or over, with only tolerable results in controlling other symptoms, but never breaking in but little upon those above given, excepting once, for a few weeks, getting a very decided action of Causticum 1,000 in relieving the constipation, she was one day seized with an acute pain just under the left axilla, which darted from there horizontally across the chest into the right lung, and with it came also darting pains in the upper half of both lungs, and shooting from there up into the throat, and sometimes to behind both ears. For these pains we prescribed Calcarea carbonicum 6,000, one dose, which in a few hours fully subdued them all, and since that, now two weeks, she has shown more gain in the whole condition than she has before under any remedy.

SPIGELIA.

The acute pains of this drug, illustrated on plate No. 4, by three arrows starting out from one circle beneath the left mamma, and extending, one to the left shoulder, another to the left scapula, and a third into the sternum, we have confirmed in the following case: June 2, 1870, we were called to an unmarried lady aged twenty-eight years, who, upon examination was found to be laboring under an attack of acute rheumatic inflammation of the heart. The bellows murmur was loud and distinct. In the previous six or eight years she said she had had two very severe attacks of inflammatory rheumatism, and both times treated with local applications. But this time, as was to have been expected from the former suppressing treatment, the disease seized at once upon the heart, and soon developed acute pains through the præcordial region. We at first administered Aconite 1,000, expecting it would subdue the inflammatory condition, but as it did not in twenty-four hours, and the pains were becoming more severe, we prescribed Bryonia 2,000. Ten hours later we were summoned to our patient in great haste, and found her in apparently the most excruciating agony, from acute pains in the left chest. She could scarcely take an inspiration, and could not even move hand or foot, so great were the aggravations therefrom. Upon inquiry, the pain was ascertained to start from the region of the apex of the heart, and shoot, one branch to the left shoulder and down the front and inside of the left upper arm, another branch backward and upward to about the center of the left scapula, and a third branch from left to right into the lower extremity of the sternum. Pulse 140 per minute. We then gave Spigelia 1,000 one dose, and it certainly did not exceed half an hour, before great relief from all the symptoms was afforded. After this, as auscultation showed constant improvement in the sounds of the heart and the whole condition there, we administered no more medicine for four days, though there was some pain most of the time, and occasionally very severe threatening of a return of the acute suffering, but this would soon pass over again, until the fourth day, when there was no more evidence of a cessation of the improvement, and we gave another dose of Spigelia 1,000. This again relieved for three days, though not as much as at first, when the symptoms called more prominently for Bryonia, one dose of which we gave in the 200th potency, and from that on no more medicine was needed to fully restore her to health in two or three weeks. While the heart was improving, considerable rheumatic action showed itself in the right thumb, right elbow and right ankle, and some also in the left knee and left ankle; but for this we did nothing, allowing the above named remedies to complete the whole cure, as has already been stated that they did.

BORAX VENETA.

The following is the confirmation by Dr. Kenyon, of the symptom of Borax, illustrated by an arrow extending from before backward beneath the right clavicle, through the apex of the right lung. The patient was an unmarried lady aged twenty-eight, and her case here follows: The doctor was first called to her for an attack of acute sore throat, and says: Upon examination he found the entire fauces, as far down as he could see, completely covered with whitish pimples, strewn as thickly together as they could stand. There was extreme suffering from deglutition, and great burning sensation in the fauces, extending down the throat. Mercurius corrosivus relieved these symptoms promptly, but two or three days following, some other throat symptoms manifested themselves, for which he prescribed Baryta carbonicum. This appeared to control all remaining troubles, and he heard nothing more from his patient for four or five weeks, when he was called again and found her complaining of burning and raw feeling in the fauces, and oppressed respiration. This was in February, 1869, and these symptoms continued, with but little, if any relief from various remedies, until the last of May, when there arose an acute or *sharp aching pressure* just beneath the right clavicle, and extending through to the right scapula. After the appearance of this symptom, there was still no curative action established by medicine, through the summer, and no time that she would pass more than a week or ten days without an increase of the symptoms of soreness and burning in the throat, or an aggravation of the acute pain under the clavicle, until December, when there appeared a glandular swelling in the left axilla. For a time this was very painful, remaining about the same for four weeks, then, under the action of Lycopodium, suppuration took place rapidly, and entire relief followed, both to the throat symptoms, and the pain through the apex of the lung for another four weeks. The pain then returned, but not the sore throat, and continued until February 20, 1870, when, acting upon the statement as to the action of Borax upon the upper right lung, he administered one dose of Borax 3,000. The result was an immediate subsidence of the pain, and the evening following, the moment she laid down, there arose a sensation as though she were *falling out of bed*, and during the night she dreamed much of falling out of bed, and would wake with a start. The sense of falling, and the dreams, persisted in returning for several successive nights, but there was no return of pain or throat symptoms until March 7th, fifteen days, when there was a slight recurrence of the pain, and another dose of Borax 3,000 was given, followed with a repetition of all the sensations and dreams of falling out of bed. After this there was no further pain until the middle of May, when it arose again in a good deal of severity. Borax 3000, one dose, was again prescribed, with the identical sensation of falling, but each time the dream was less. The pain did not return until August 19th, and then but slightly, when Borax 3000 was again repeated, but as she has been absent on a visit, the result has not yet been learned. In addition to the Borax he also gave three doses of Arum triphyllum 5000, the first one June 22, 1870, and the other two at intervals of two or three weeks, for burning and a sense of excoriation of the fauces and a husky, changeable voice, which then arose for the first time in some six months, and this drug afforded quick relief, each time, to these symptoms.

A still further important fact and result with the patient was, that she had had an attack of "Hay-fever" between the 10th of June, and July 1st, every summer for nine years in succession, until this summer, when there was no appearance of it, thus showing that this disease, as well as the other symptoms of the case had been broken up by the treatment.

Since writing the above we received the following note from Dr. Kenyon in regard to the case, and the result of the last dose of Borax.

"DEAR DOCTOR:—My patient has returned and has had no recurrence of either sore throat, or the pain under the right clavicle; and says she has ridden over rough roads, and exercised in various other ways, that she knows would heretofore have excited both, for frequently, getting into a street car and riding a few blocks, would bring on the pain very severely. L. M. K."

According to this result, the arrow illustrating that symptom of Borax, should have had the character representing pressure, upon it, to correspond with the sensation of *sharp aching pressure*, a fact we did not know when the illustration was made.

CANTHARIS AND ZINCUM METALLICUM.

"I have had two cases where the medicine acted like a charm, and produced relief in a few minutes. One was a case of sticking pain in the chest, just above the region of the heart, and flying both ways, not affected by inspiration, shooting to the sternum and axilla, left side: Cantharis.

"The other was a lady who had been suffering from ulceration of the cervex uteri, and has lately had a tumor removed. The pain began at the pit of the stomach, and would pass up following the course of the œsophagus, with a sense of drawing, and a cold streak; it afterward changed to a gurgling sensation, but was removed both times by Zincum metallicum. BLAKELY."

Although these cases are given so briefly, yet how important they become. Think of it; a physician is led by an illustrated symptom, to at once, and without hesitation, select and prescribe, the *only* known *curative* remedy in the world, for that symptom, which had arisen probably, in the second case certainly, from a serious diseased condition of the system, and finds the medicine acting "like a charm," and giving "relief in a *few minutes*." Can anything be more astounding than such results in a field where we have all, no doubt, been too much given to view matters in the light of doubt and uncertainty? That the picture is not overdrawn by the doctor, we fully believe, for we have, ourselves, seen just astonishing results, and point to the next case as a sample of many such that have come under our observation.

COCCULUS.

August 25, 1870, we were called to a man aged forty-six,

who, after passing through the premonitory symptoms, for two or three weeks, was, the day before our call, taken down with typhoid fever. The symptom of which he complained the most was a *dull aching pain* through the forehead, and from there back to the center of the head, it not being felt much in the temples. This was controlled in two or three days, and the appearances were that the fever was being broken, but a day or two following that, the same kind of pain seated in the abdomen, just below the umbilicus, and increased in severity from day to day, notwithstanding the administration of Nux vomica, Rhus toxicodendron, etc., until, in a few days, it culminated in a very acute pain, darting through just below the umbilicus to the spine. For that we prescribed Belladonna, Bryonia, and Pulsatilla in succession, giving each one day to develop its effect, but without any relief, and then allowed ourselves to be governed especially by this one symptom of acute pain, without reference to the other indications of the case, and gave Cocculus, according to the illustration of it on plate 3, though this drug seemed so foreign to our patient's condition, in all else excepting that pain. The next day we found that all acute suffering had ceased, leaving the same aching pain and a soreness behind, but it was a matter of great question with us whether the symptom had not stopped of itself, from the length of time it had continued, or if medicine had anything to do with its disappearance. Following this, the dull aching continued, and increased in severity, until it caused great suffering, and then extended into and through both legs, the right the worst, down into the great toes. And now a moderate drawing and severe bruised sensation set in with the aching, and extended to the back and into the legs, and the bowels became very much constipated. Pulse about 100 per minute, urine very turbid.

Again we prescribed Nux vomica, Rhus toxicodendron, Sulphur, and two or three other remedies, but they had no effect whatever in allaying the pain, though the tongue cleared up under their action, and all appearances of fever, and the typhoid condition wholly subsided, leaving the pain still worse, if anything, and the patient very weak. He then passed some five or six days entirely without fever, but with no abatement of pain, when a sister came from a distance to see him, and said she knew how to treat "nooraligy," and without waiting to consult us in regard to it, went to making applications of cloths wrung out of hot water, to the abdomen and limbs. The effect was decided, to say the least, for the pain was relieved in a few hours, but at our visit the next morning we found him with quite a high fever, the tongue covered with a brown coating through the center, and many other symptoms indicating a return of the whole typhoid state. Prohibiting further interference we prescribed Phosphorus, following it in a day or two with Rhus, which subdued the fever in four or five days, but no sooner had this been done than the same kind of pain returned to the abdomen, and soon became worse than at all before. He now, too, presented more indications of exhaustion of the vital energies, than at any previous time, and through it all extreme constipation continued, once going ten days without a fecal evacuation. The abdomen did not become very sensitive to pressure, from the pain, neither did it become in the least hardened, nor but slightly tympanitic.

We diagnosed the case as one in which the suffering arose from diseased action, or irritation, in the spinal cord, having passed down the spine from the brain under the effect of medicine the first few days, and that the pain in the abdomen and legs was the result of the nerves manifesting their sufferings at their extremities in those parts. But what was to cure this condition, was the more important question? We now again tried Nux vomica, Belladonna, Pulsatilla, Bryonia and Rhus toxicodendron, then Mercurius, Colocynth, and Veratrum, but each day he suffered more, groaning every breath when awake, and not sleeping to exceed two or three hours in twenty-four, then only from sheer exhaustion, until most profuse *cold* perspiration set in, and finally one day when we called, indications of paralysis of the organs of deglutition had arisen, though there had not before been the slightest suffering of any kind in those parts. He had no appetite, in fact, a great repugnance to food of all kinds, but we had ordered beef tea, etc., and insisted upon his eating something, so that morning he tried to eat a piece of toast, but in attempting to swallow, the throat would not act at all to pass it down into the œsophagus, and after three or four efforts he had to desist. Pulse was now running to about 130 per minute; hands very cold and becoming purple.

In reflecting upon our patient's condition, it did not seem to us possible that he could live to exceed two days, if he was not relieved in a few hours. So, from not knowing what better to do, and more in a fit of despair than from the exercise of any skill, we put together the two facts of the darting pain below the umbilicus through to the spine, which had arisen in the early stage of the case, and the threatening paralysis of the fauces, or œsophagus, which had now come up, and upon these two symptoms prescribed Cocculns 1,000, one dose, followed by Saccharum lactis. Making an appointment to visit him again in a few hours, we left, with scarcely a ray of hope ever seeing him any better. But at the next visit, some eight hours later, almost the whole condition of the patient had changed or was rapidly changing. His wife said that it was not more than fifteen or twenty minutes after we gave him the dose of medicine, before he called for toast and ate a whole slice of it with evident relish, and without any difficulty in swallowing. The cold perspiration, which had been very profuse the night before and that morning, had almost wholly ceased, the pain had so far subsided that there was no more groaning, nor a complaint of it, though upon inquiry he said he still felt it slightly; his voice, which had been very weak was now quite strong, in short, he seemed in all respects like another man. He slept well the night following, and the next day found him almost without symptoms, except the debility, which was, of course, very great, but he rallied rapidly from this, his bowels became regular in their action, the appetite good, and we dismissed him ten days after, able to walk out of doors a short distance, and not requiring further medical attendance. Such, then, as extreme as it may seem, was all the result of the action of *one dose* of Cocculus 1,000, for we did not give him another dose of it after the one mentioned. The improvement was so rapid that it would have been the height of folly to have meddled in any way with it, even by one more dose of the same remedy.

Now, is it not clear, that Cocculus was the only drug indicated in this case, *first, last, and all the time* (it has: "*Aching pain in the forehead*," the first prominent symptom of the patient), while all the other remedies given were useless, or, perhaps, worse than useless? And had we allowed ourselves to have been governed by the *one* symptom of acute pain darting through the abdomen, below the umbilicus, to the spine, as we had illustrated this on plate 3, and held to this remedy from that time, should we not have cured our patient without ever allowing a dangerous symptom to have arisen, and avoided all the extreme suffering? And if so, do we go too far in saying that the exact locality, direction, and extent of any specific kind of pain is of far more consequence, because more characteristic as guides in therapeutics, than all else besides in any case of disease where pains locate themselves, and remain long enough to show there is no doubt about them. From our experience thus far in this matter, we are led to place just as much reliance upon the locality and direction of aching, boring, burning, drawing, pinching, pressing, throbbing, and other pains, as true guides in the indications of remedies, as we do upon the darting or stitching pains.

In conclusion, we will say we firmly believe that highly attenuated medicines are capable of *always* performing as remarkable cures, or nearly so, as Cocculus did in this instance, while disease remains *functional*, or before it reaches the point of developing organic changes, and where its primary causes are not daily or frequently renewed, as in sufferings brought on by errors in diet, or other abuses; and the only reason why physicians of our school do not uniformly get such effects, is from our not yet having the means of always positively knowing the one and only specific remedy indicated in every case, then relying upon that, and avoiding its too frequent repetition. Let us all, then, work together in this promising field, and have every symptom of every drug illustrated as soon as possible, so that we shall have that great aid, before unused, to the knowledge we need.

RHUS RADICANS.

One day last summer, the draughtsman who has made the drawing for all our illustrations, came in and said he was taken that morning on rising, with a "drawing and stitching pain," which started in at the left nipple, and extended through to the left scapula. There was no cough, nor other symptoms, but the pain had gradually increased in severity, he said, until then, when it was causing severe suffering, and his countenance was quite pale. One dose of Rhus radicans 200 was given, which relieved him entirely in from one to two hours, and he has never had this symptom since.

CONIUM.

We recently received the following highly interesting and concisely reported case, from Dr. L. Shafer "In the Illustrated Repertory, you say, Conium also has: 'Violent stitches in the side, as if a knife were plunged into the side, causing loud moaning.' 'Whether right or left, or both sides, is not here designated, so we place the arrow upon each side, and leave the matter for further confirmation or correction."

"The following may throw some light upon the subject, so far as the right side is concerned:

"In February, 1870, was called to see Mrs. ——, aged seventy-five. Found her laboring under a severe attack of pneumonia, affecting her right lung. The respirations were somewhat accelerated and painful, the cough troublesome, the sputa rust-colored, the tongue coated and whitish, the pulse about 100. Under the use of Aconite 200, followed by Bryonia 30, the symptoms were considerably mitigated. On calling again I found a marked change in the symptoms. She complained of 'violent stitches in the side, as if a knife were plunged into the side, causing loud moaning.' On inquiry as to the precise situation of the pain, she pointed out, upon her person, exactly the region covered by the arrow on the right side in plate 1.

" A few pellets of Conium 30, were dissolved in a dozen teaspoonfuls of water, and a teaspoonful ordered to be given every three hours. The pain soon passed off, as by magic, and the patient made a rapid and very satisfactory recovery."

Does not the above prove that the one symptom of stitches in the locality named was of far more value than all the other symptoms of the case combined? Who would have otherwise thought of Conium as a curative remedy in pneumonia, and given it in preference to several other remedies for *rust-colored sputa*? And yet we see that under it, " *the pain passed off, as by magic*," and the " patient made a *rapid* recovery," of course from *all* other symptoms as well as the pain.

INDEX.

R

S

T

V

Z

Spotted something that isn't quite right?

Let us know and we'll fix it for future reprints.
And as a thank you for your diligence, we'll
send you a free Sothis book of your choice.

publisher@sothis.press

This page intentionally left blank

Made in United States
Orlando, FL
05 November 2026

90296041R00062